The Lighter Side of YOGA

by Mike Nevitt
Foreword by Danny Paradise

SANTA
MONICA
PRESS

Published by: Santa Monica Press LLC
P.O. Box 850
Solana Beach, CA 92075
1-800-784-9553
www.santamonicapress.com
books@santamonicapress.com

SANTA
MONICA
PRESS

Printed in the United States

Santa Monica Press books are available at special quantity discounts when purchased in bulk
by corporations, organizations, or groups. Please call our Special Sales department at 1-800-784-9553.

ISBN-13 978-1-59580-109-8

Cover and interior design and production by Future Studio

Follow The Lighter Side of Yoga on Facebook and Instagram

For Hanne, Butterfly, and little Scruffy

All the great masters and teachers of yoga and meditation had two things in common: great humility and great humor. I'm very happy to write the foreword for this book as it is plainly evident that when people take the practices and teachings of yoga too seriously, we see those practices become heavy and lacking in the element of lightness that contributes to the awakenings and freedoms that the practices offer.

I consider yoga to be the science of happiness and healing, the science of breath, flexibility, balance, and strength, and very significantly—the science of aging well. With all this it's not surprising that yoga has become a global phenomenon with people on all continents and from different races and cultures enjoying the benefits of the practice.

My own explorations in yoga began in 1976 with the first western adepts of Ashtanga yoga, David Williams and Nancy Gilgoff. They were in the lineage of the Indian Ayurvedic physician and yogi T. Krishnamacharya, who is considered today to be one of the grandfathers of contemporary yoga. Krishnamacharya taught some of the world's most renowned and influential teachers including B.K.S. Iyengar, K. Pattabhi Jois, Indra Devi, and T.K.V. Desikachar. Very quickly, I realized that I was feeling better through the practice of yoga. I became stronger, more flexible, clear in my mind, more balanced, peaceful, and more aware. I began to travel the world and introduce yoga internationally in the late '70s as well as playing music and performing. Through music and serendipity I began teaching yoga to famous artists and musicians such as Sting, Madonna, Marcel Marceau, Paul Simon, Eddie Vedder, Bob Weir, Luciano Pavarotti, and others.

Mike Nevitt has been a longtime student and friend of mine. I first met him in 1996 during a two-week retreat I was leading in Oxford, England. After years of dedicated practice, he became a gifted teacher in his own right, and through this book shows the depth of his experience and observations within the world of yoga over a 30-year period.

Through humor, Mike illustrates the strange, funny, occasionally crazy, and often hilarious aspects and scenarios which exist to varying degrees within the world of modern yoga.

Thank you, Mike, for your beautiful gift of seeing and sharing *The Lighter Side of Yoga*.

INTRODUCTION

This book is the culmination of 30 years of observation and experiences as a teacher of yoga and meditation. It wasn't planned; it sprang spontaneously into existence one day in 2017 with a cartoon scribble I posted online which received a large number of likes and comments. Over the years I had become more and more disillusioned with the yoga world and what was happening within it. Due to an explosive trend of teacher training programs being offered by yoga studios, there was soon a saturation of new yoga teachers everywhere and this was accompanied by the appearance of online companies offering free exposure to studios and teachers in exchange for half-price deals and other incentives. I felt the authenticity and depth of yoga was disappearing.

I did a second cartoon, which also received a great deal of attention, and much of the feedback was from people instantly relating to the message of the cartoon, which depicted a character disturbing a room full of people in Savasana by answering a call on his mobile phone.

It was inspiring and I realized that from the experiences I'd had during my decades of teaching, I actually had hundreds of these little cartoons inside me just bursting to get out!

Some of the cartoons are complete fiction,

many are from real situations and events, and others are inspired by "what if" scenarios, like the cartoon where Peter goes nuts in the meditation session and sings an Elvis number out loud. Most of the characters in the book are actually me at various stages throughout my 30-year journey as a teacher and student. I've been (and still am) Cosmic Johnny, I've been the arrogant one, the greedy one, the humble one, the lonely one, the spiritual one, the smart-ass, and the lazy one. Though most are me, I suspect and hope you might also see yourself in at least a few of the cartoons.

It's my wish with this book that the cartoons will make people laugh or induce a reflective smile, and also offer a gentle poke to remind yoga teachers and students alike not to take themselves too seriously. I hope to offer from a humorous perspective some insight into what it can actually be like to be a yoga teacher and highlight that no matter how advanced we become (whatever that means) we are all just human beings with flaws and failings working with our own journey through this wonderful practice we call yoga.

—Mike Nevitt

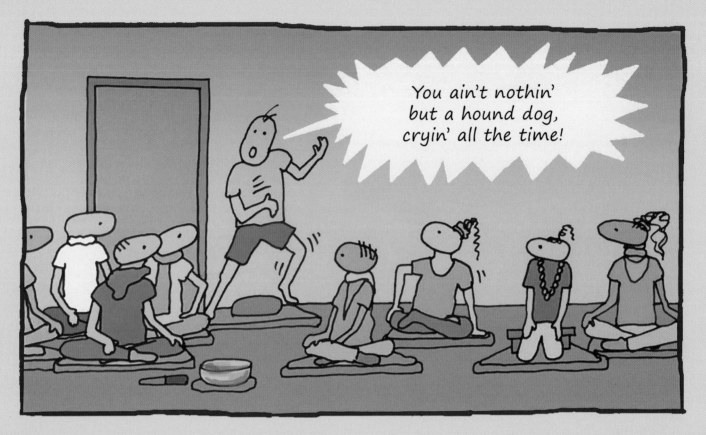

Twenty minutes into the silent meditation,
Peter suddenly went nuts.

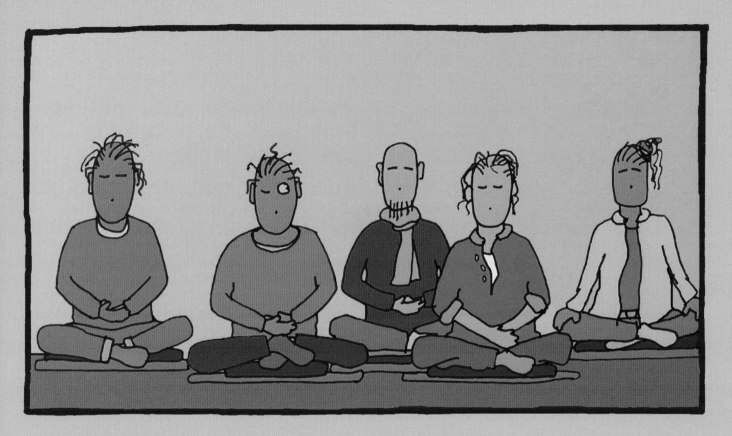

In group meditation sessions,
Tom just couldn't stop peeping.

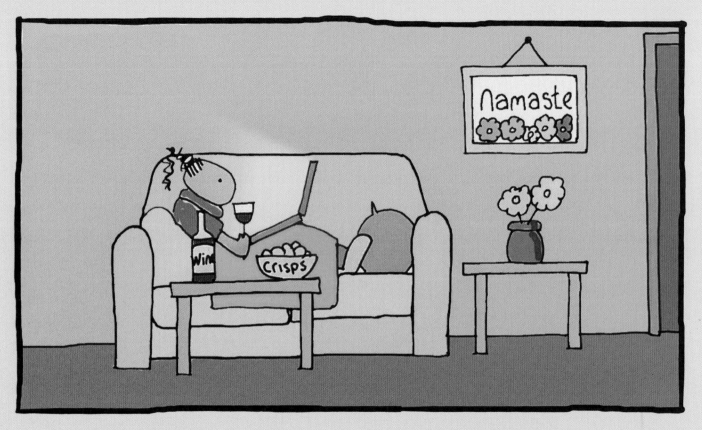

With the explosion of online yoga in Corona times,
Rachel was now attending two classes per day.

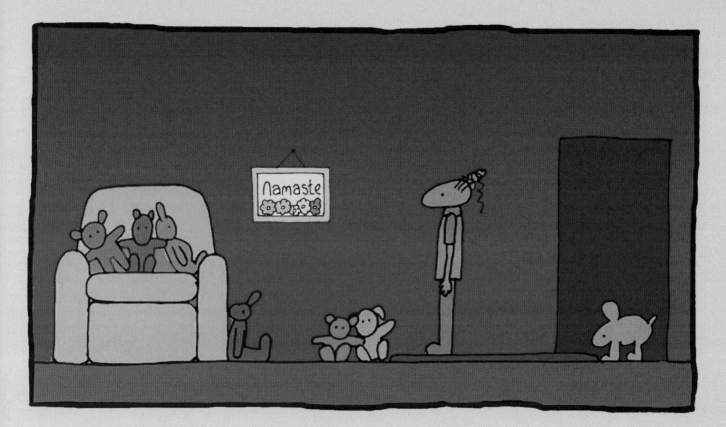

By week four of self-quarantine, Sally had more friends than ever joining in for her home yoga sessions.

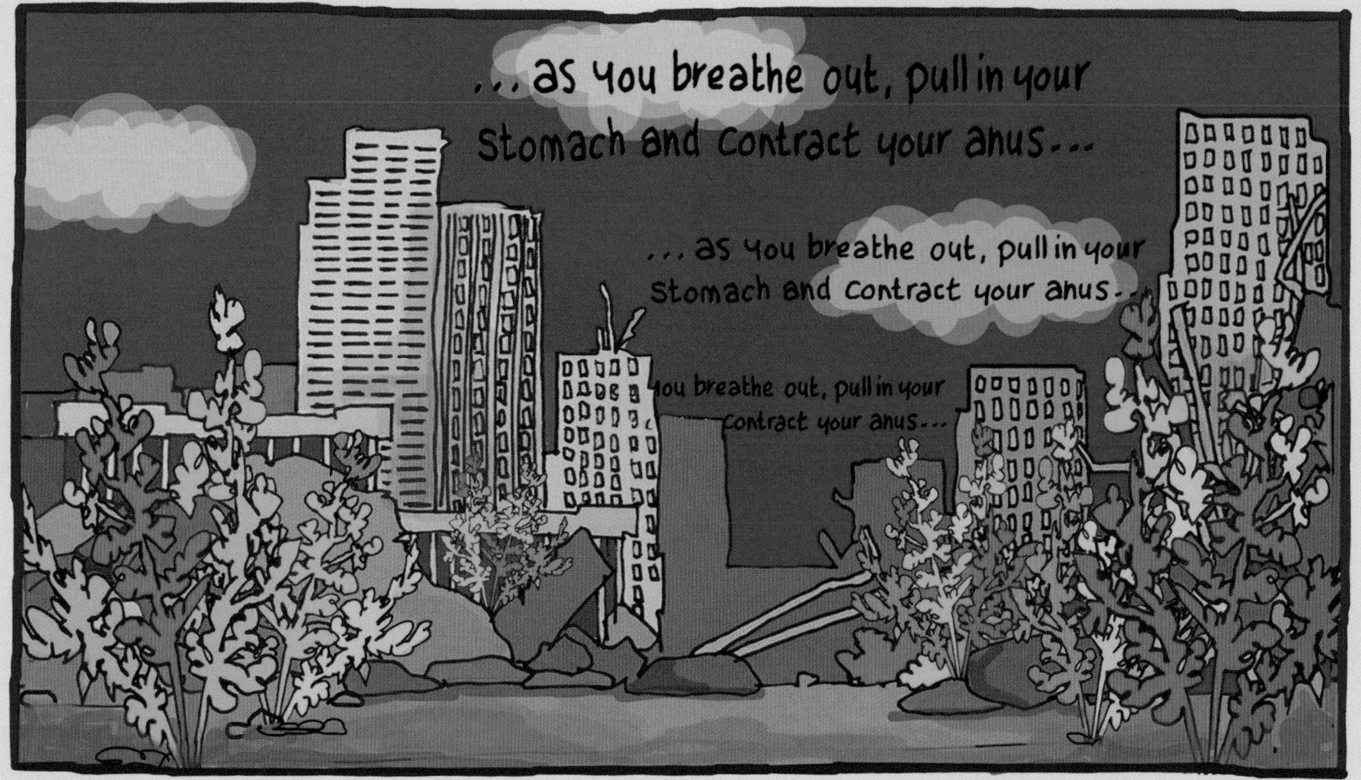
...as you breathe out, pull in your stomach and contract your anus...
...as you breathe out, pull in your stomach and contract your anus...
you breathe out, pull in your
contract your anus...

Hundreds of years into the future, a single solar-powered laptop continues to play a fragment of online yoga over and over somewhere in the abandoned city.

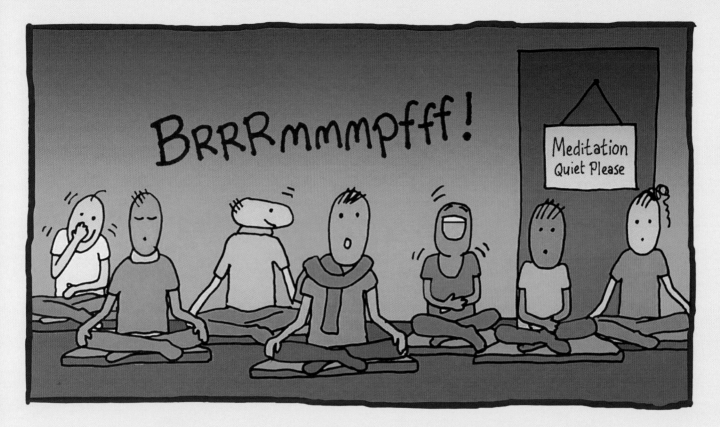

The focus of the meditation was broken somewhat
when someone in the group let out a loud, rasping ripper.

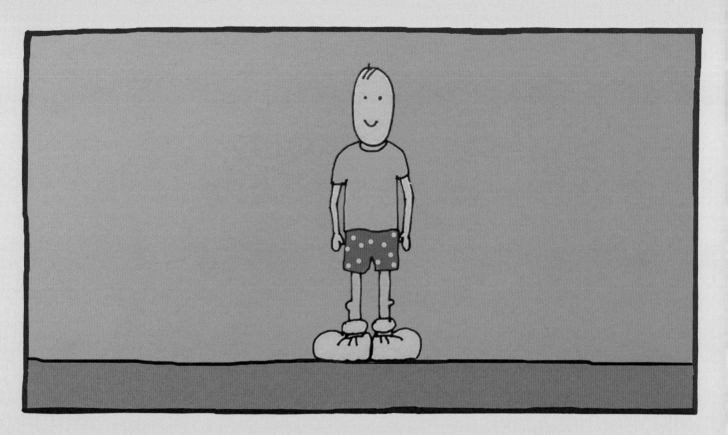

Savasana boots, one of <u>the</u> most important accessories
for any serious yoga practitioner.

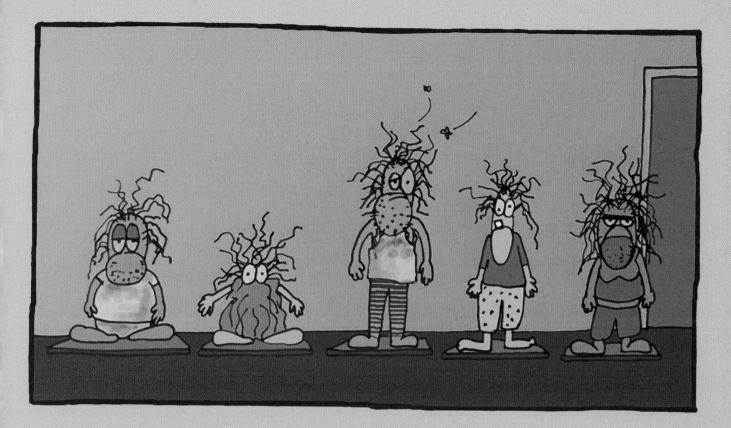

When students finally returned to live classes
after months of lockdown.

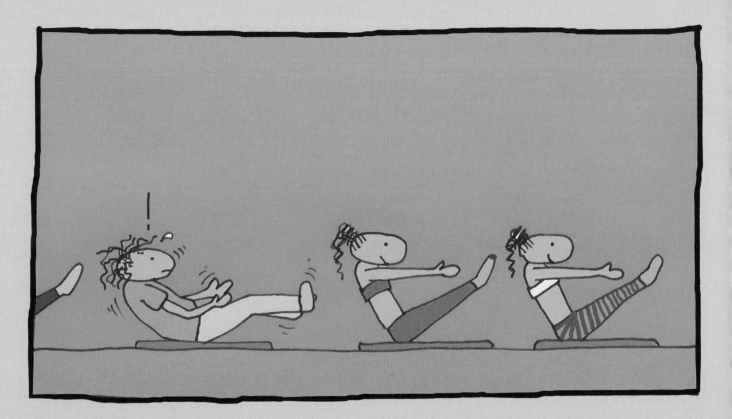

Mary was not a happy bunny, she'd mistakenly signed up for
the Navasana Challenge instead of the Savasana Challenge.

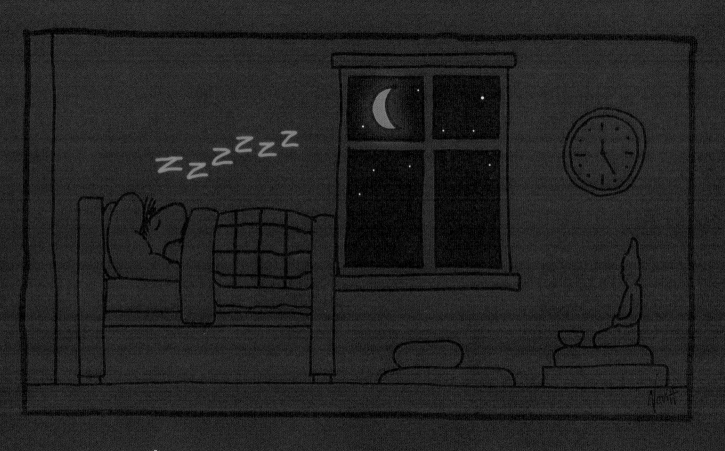

Sandra's commitment to early morning meditation sucked.

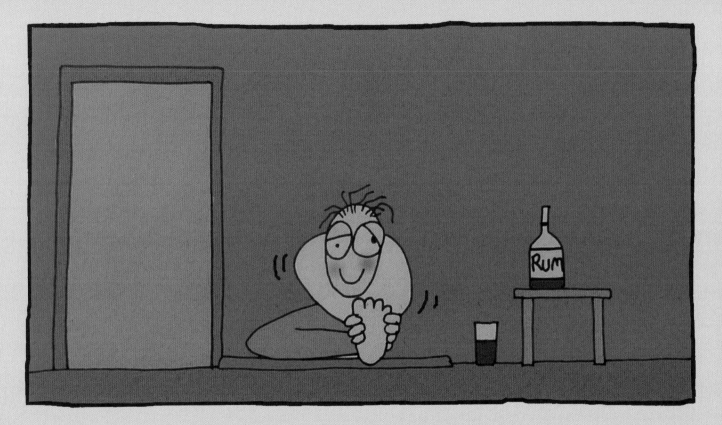

The practice just seemed to flow so much better
with Hot Rum Yoga.

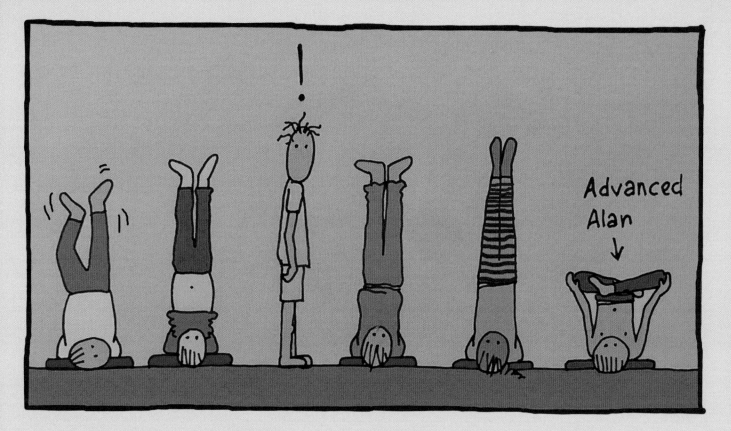

The class was going great, the sun was shining, the birds were singing, and then teacher Tom walked straight into an epic cloud of fart.

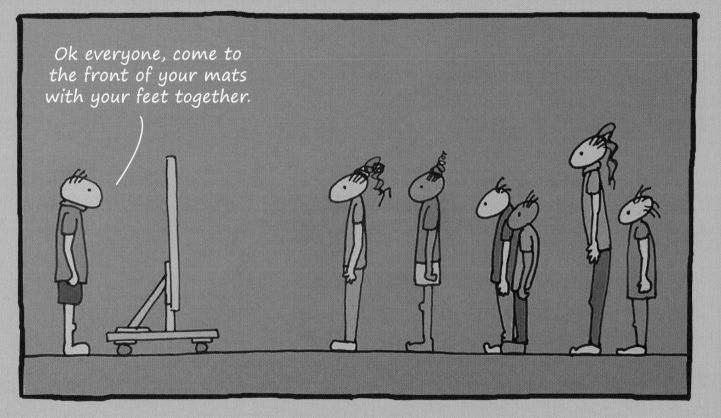

Over the years, teacher Brian had developed
an acute aversion to being stared at in class.

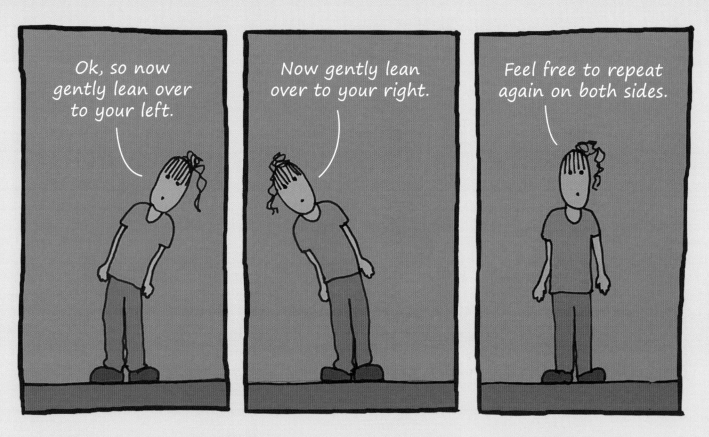

Some of the online office yoga sessions were really pushing the edge.

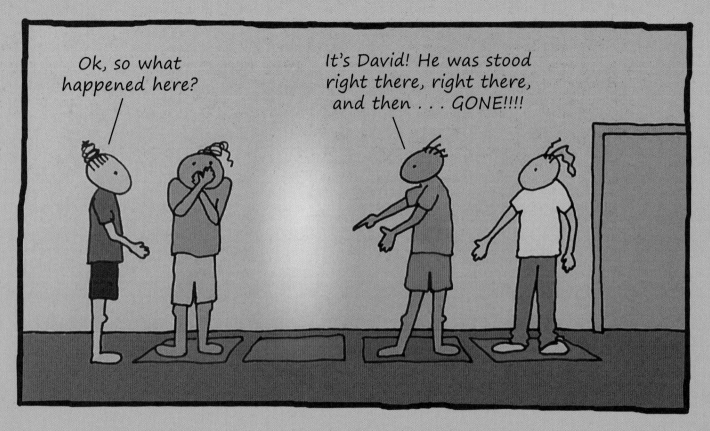

After many years of practice, David suddenly transcended his ego.

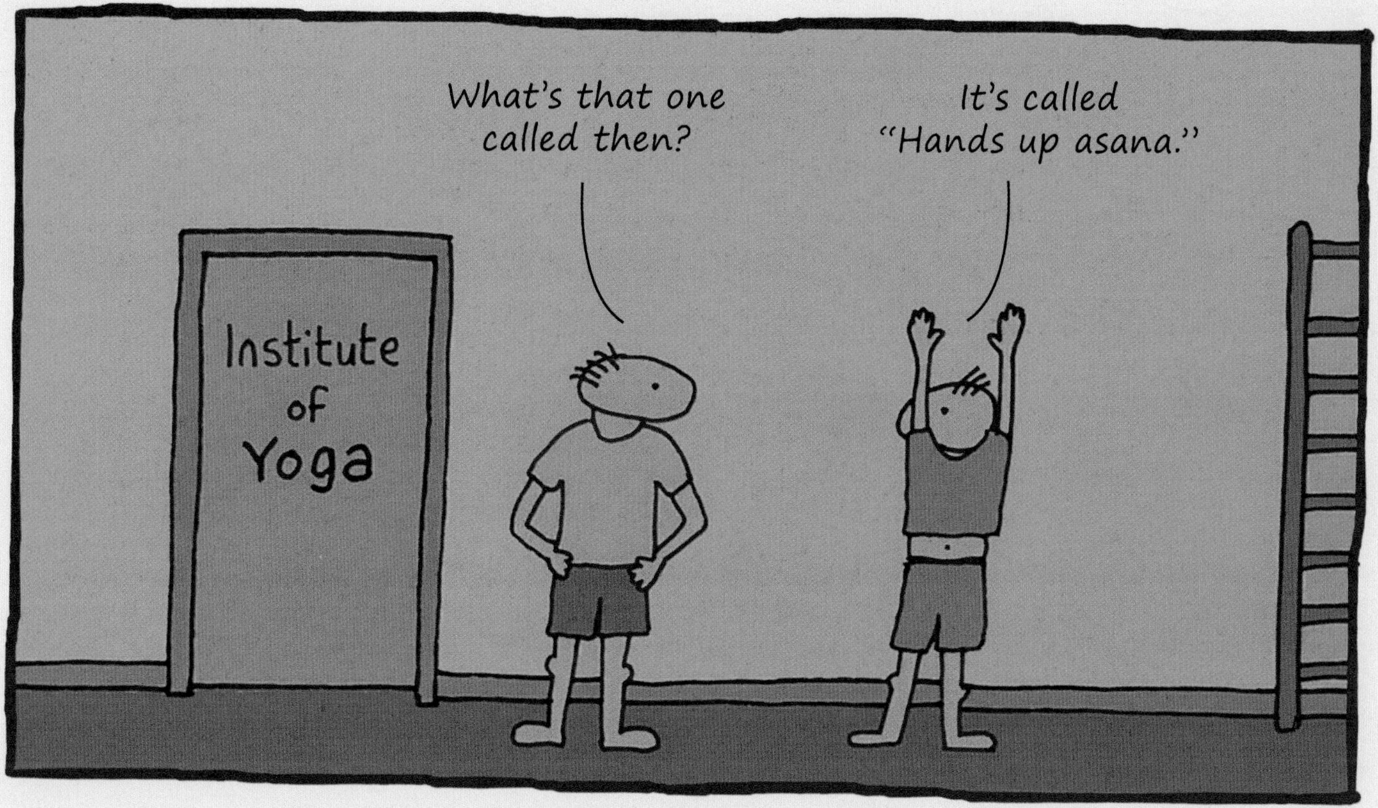
Institute of Yoga
What's that one called then?
It's called "Hands up asana."

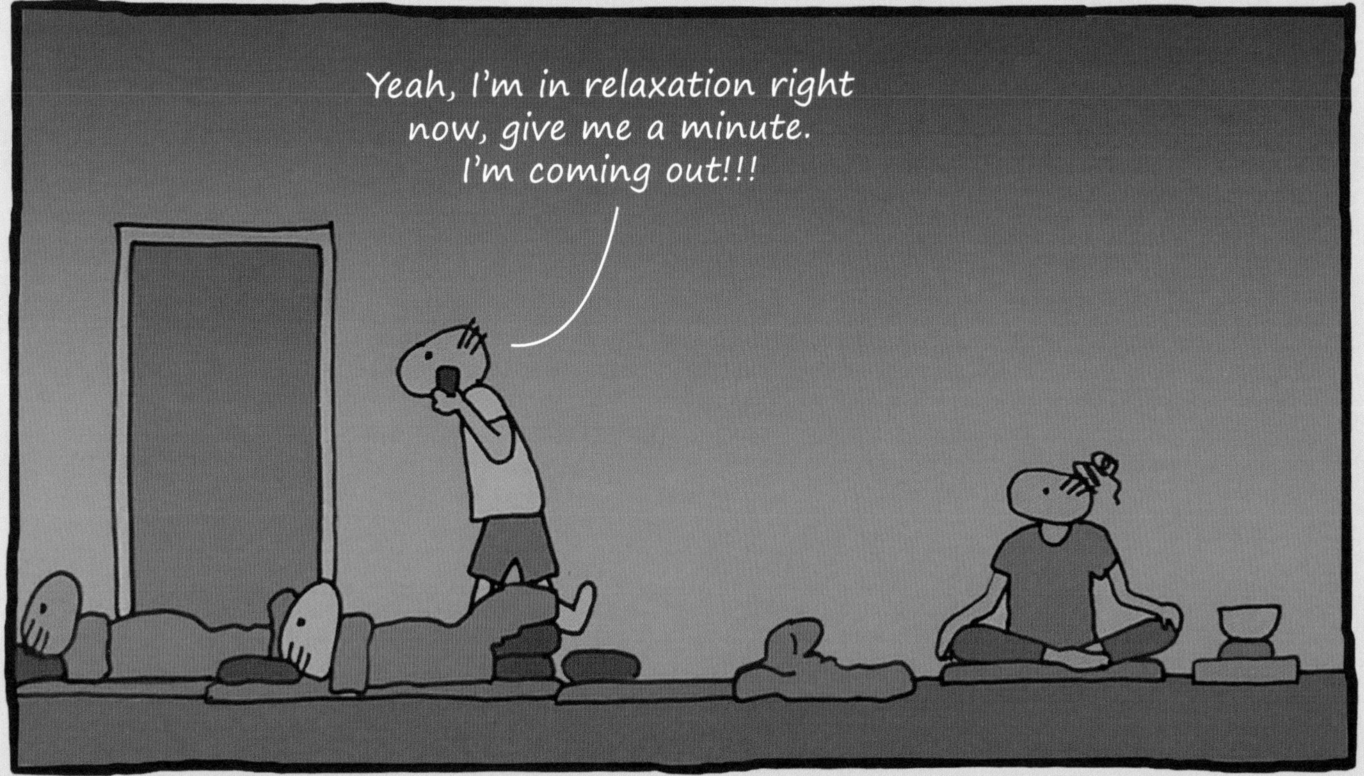
Yeah, I'm in relaxation right now, give me a minute. I'm coming out!!!

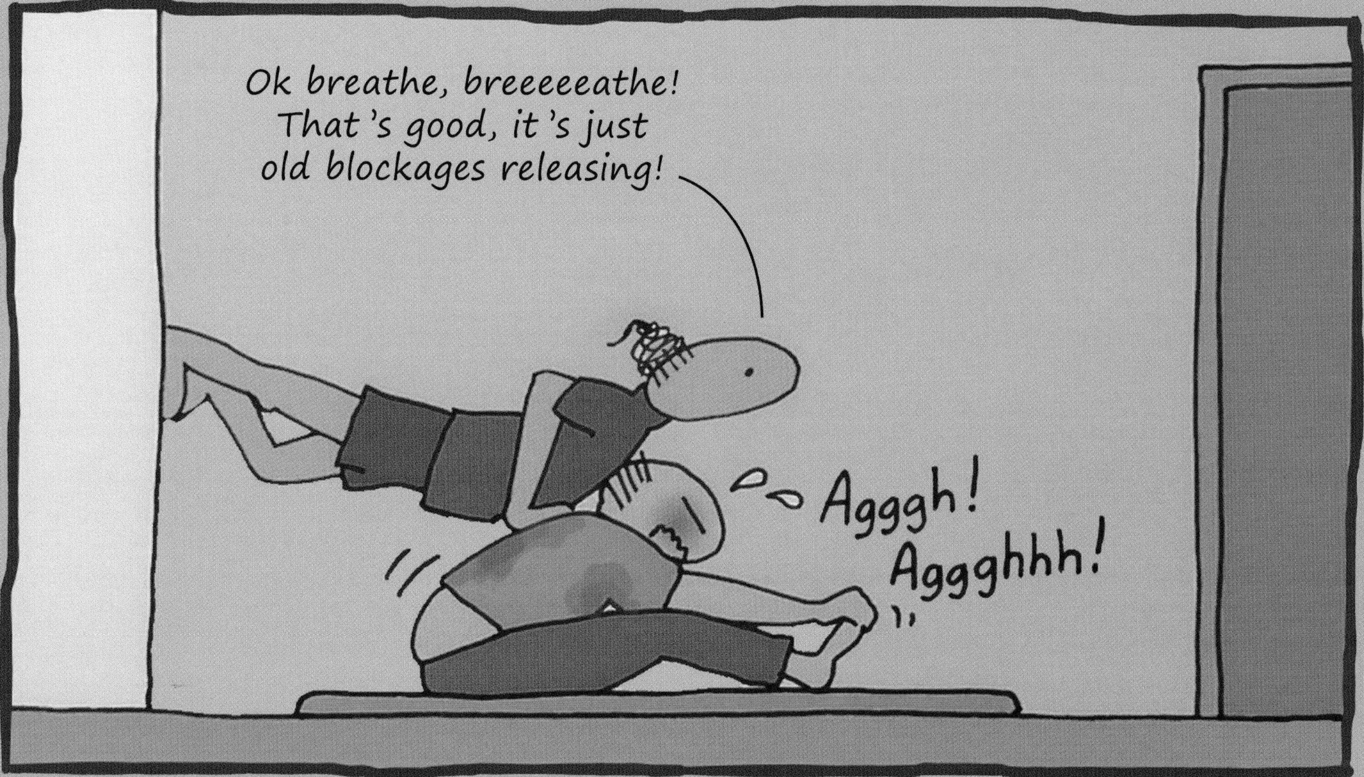
Ok breathe, breeeeeathe! That's good, it's just old blockages releasing!
Agggh!
Aggghhh!

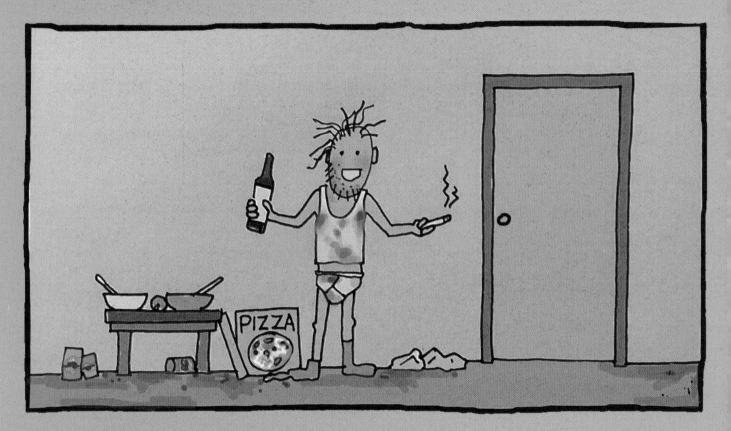

Martin's online yoga regime
had definitely begun to slip a bit recently.

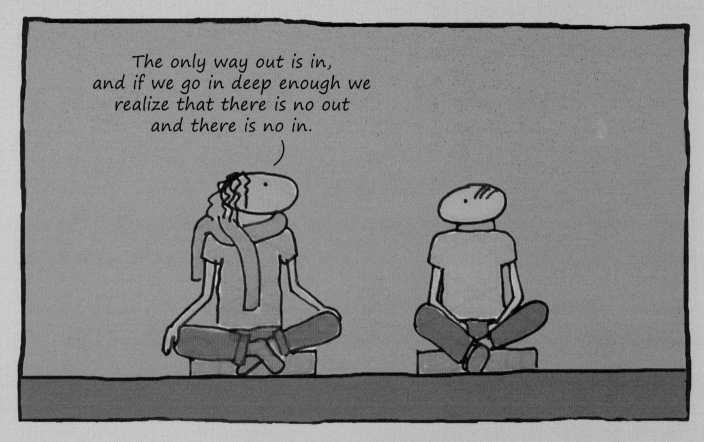

Smart asses and beginners.

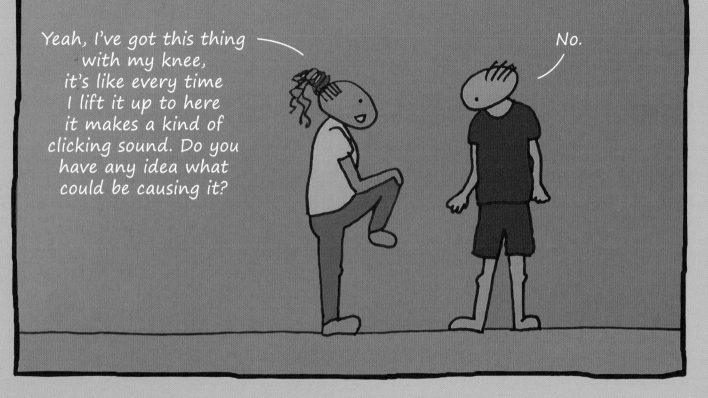

Over the years, teacher Mark had developed some pretty standard answers.

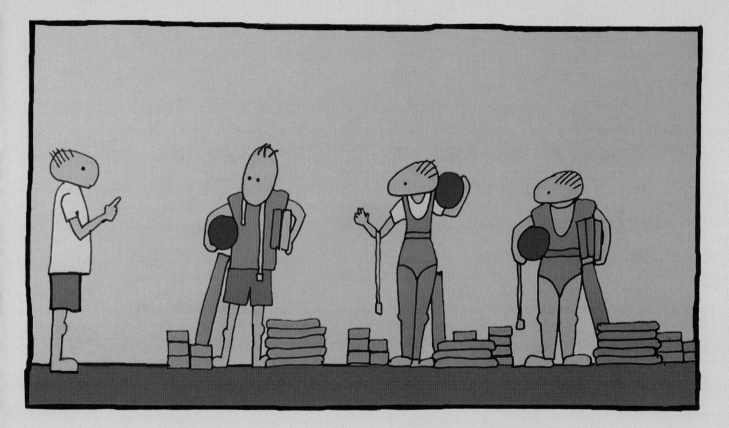

Forty minutes into the Technique Masterclass,
the students were finally ready to work on the Triangle Pose.

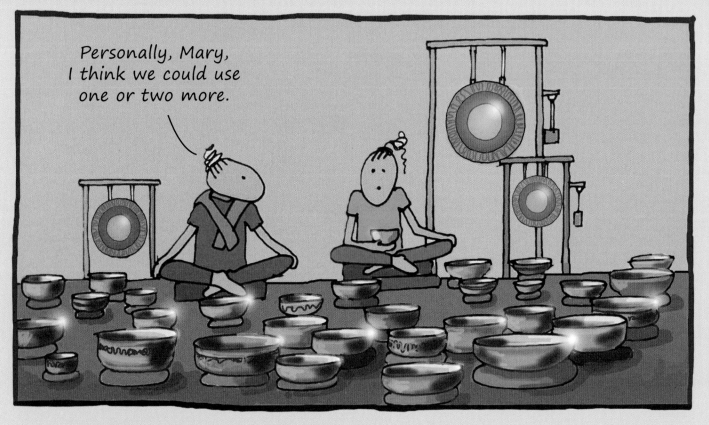

Gong night preparation.

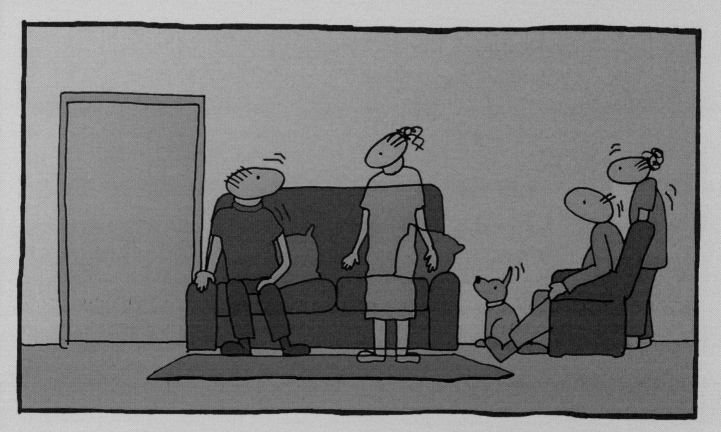

Linda had been on the Calm and Clear Meditation Intensive
for a week now and her family was becoming concerned.

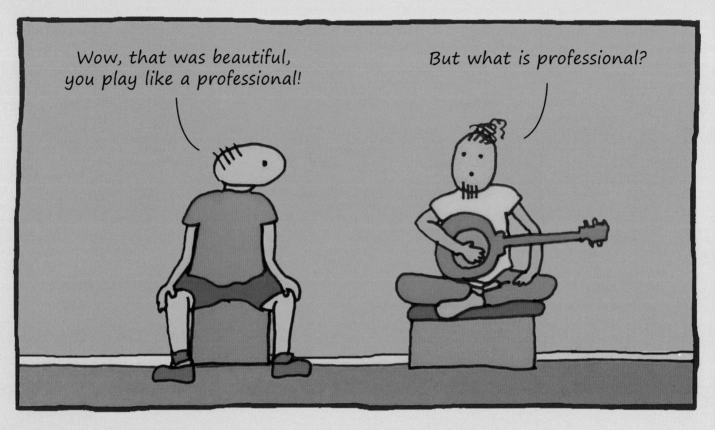

Ben was struggling to keep the conversation flowing
with the leader of the meditation retreat.

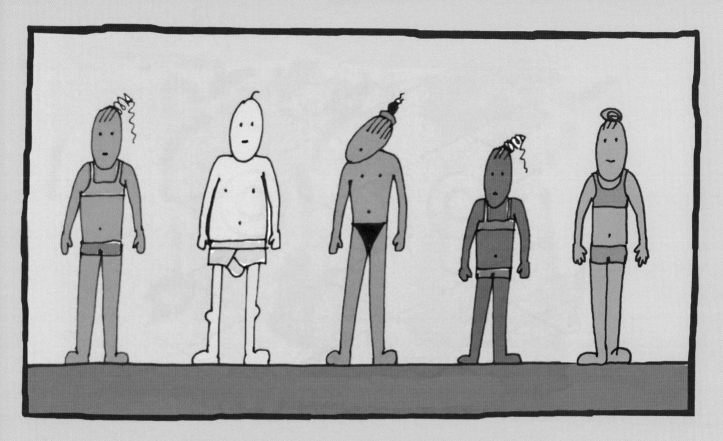

Bob's Hot Yoga outfit wasn't quite cutting it.

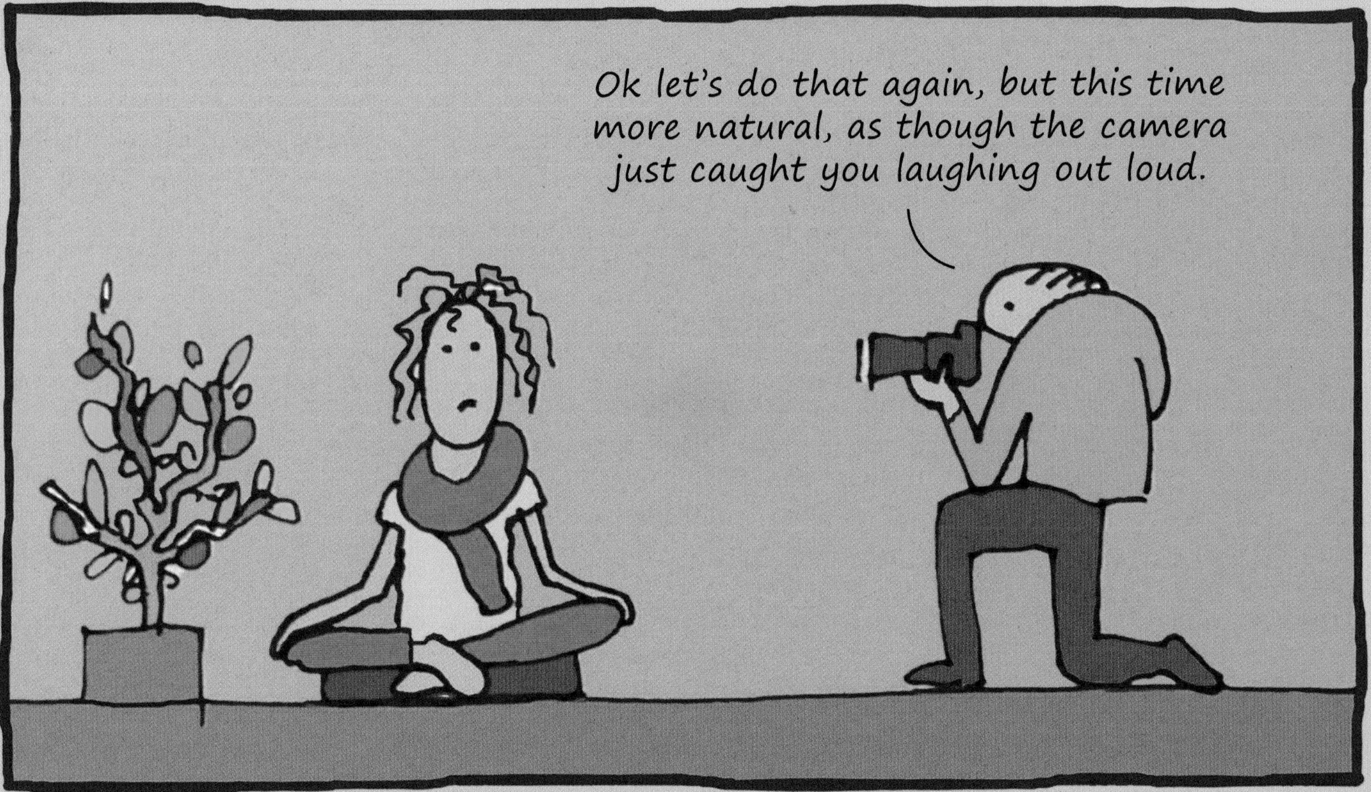
Ok let's do that again, but this time more natural, as though the camera just caught you laughing out loud.

Yoga photo sessions.

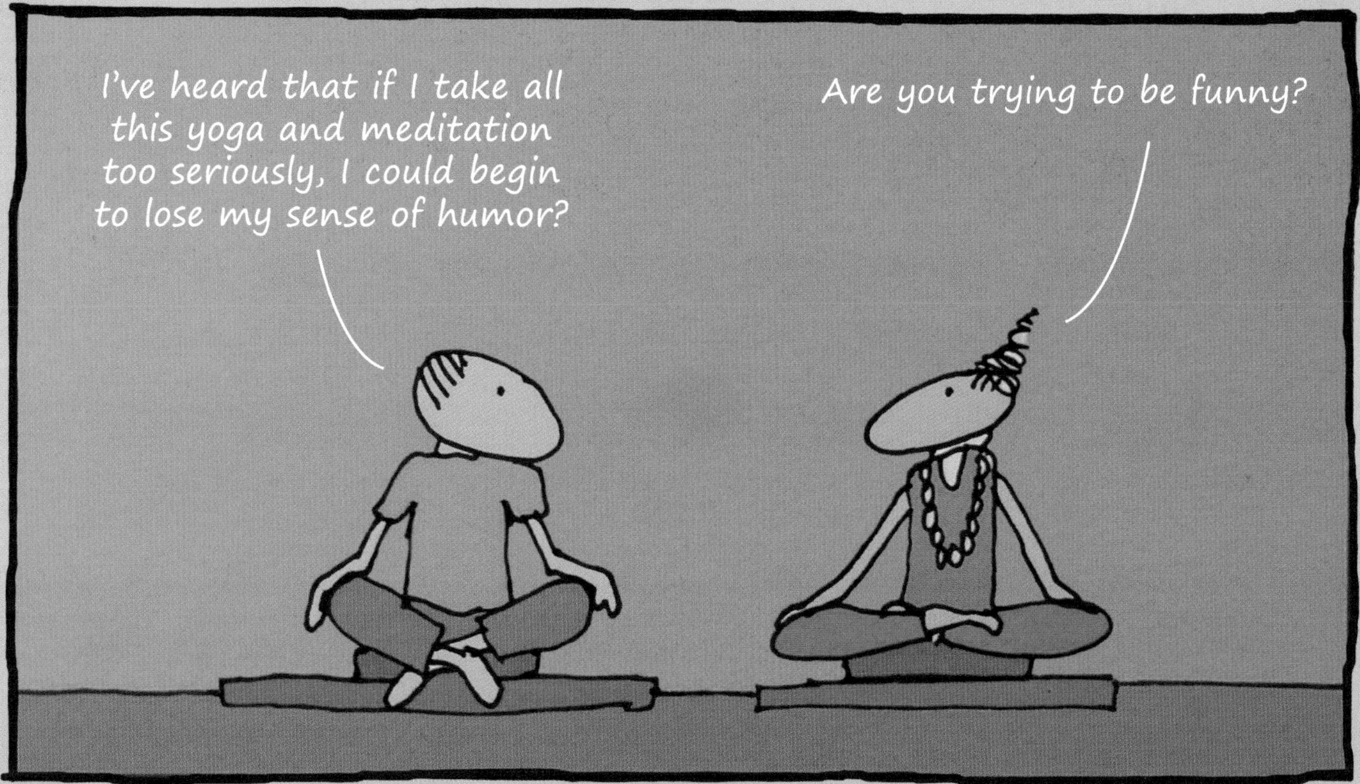
I've heard that if I take all this yoga and meditation too seriously, I could begin to lose my sense of humor?
Are you trying to be funny?

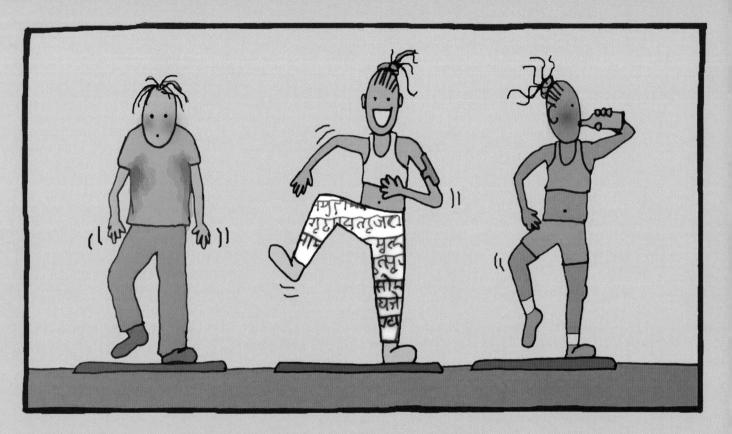

Sally's new Sanskrit leggins' were really energizing her regular workout with new depth and meaning.

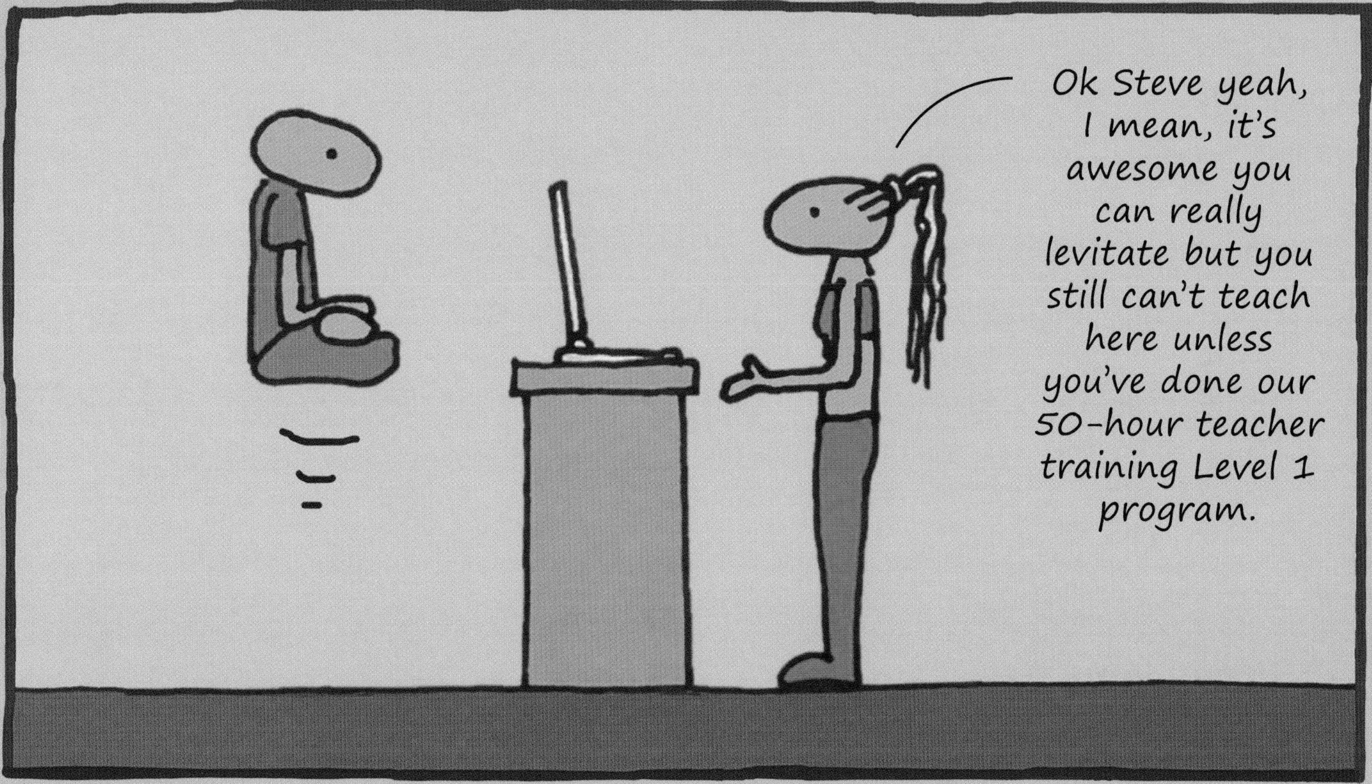
Ok Steve yeah, I mean, it's awesome you can really levitate but you still can't teach here unless you've done our 50-hour teacher training Level 1 program.

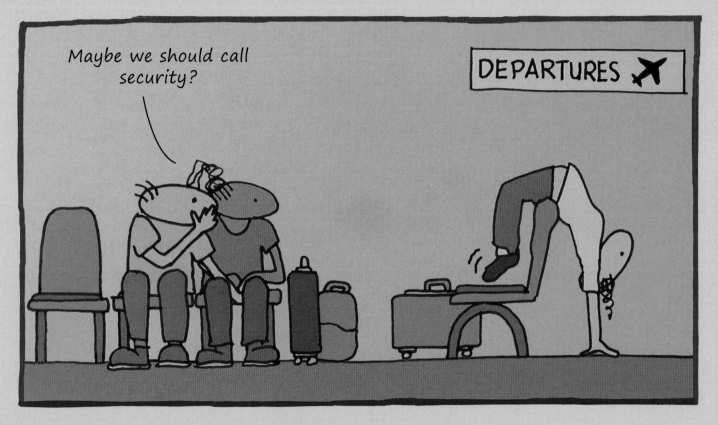

Juliet's last workshop was
"How to incorporate yoga into your everyday life."

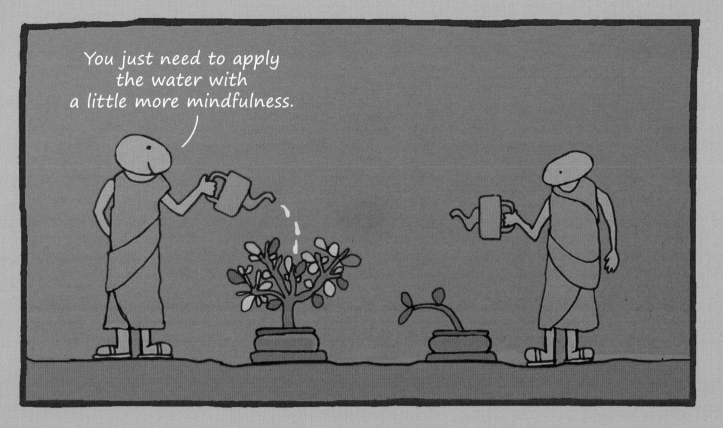

Meditation masters testing each other's egos.

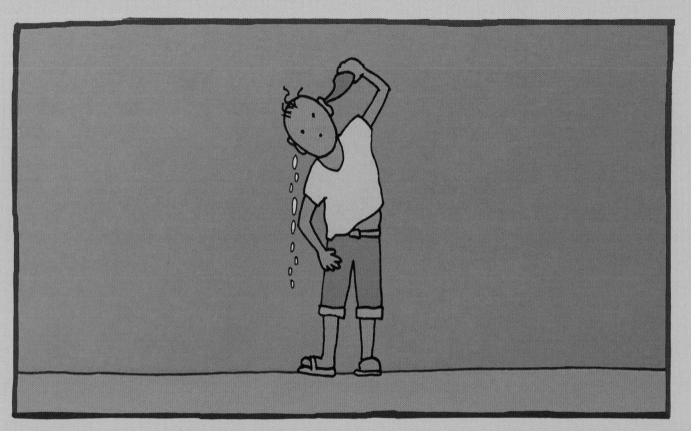

Garry had not been paying attention in the Kriya Cleansing Module during teacher training, but he did make a remarkable discovery.

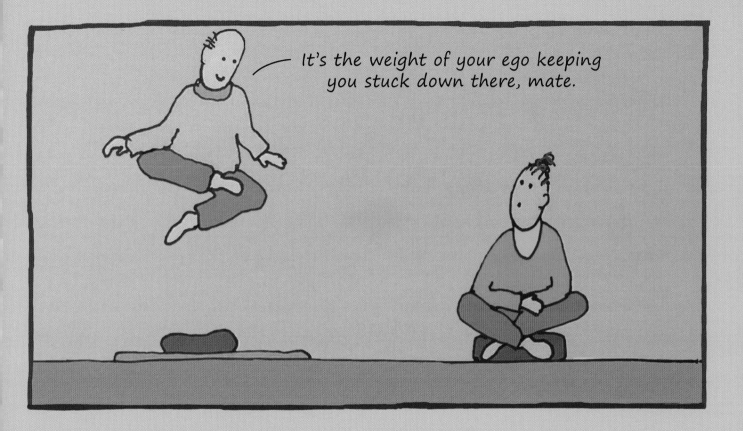

It's the weight of your ego keeping you stuck down there, mate.

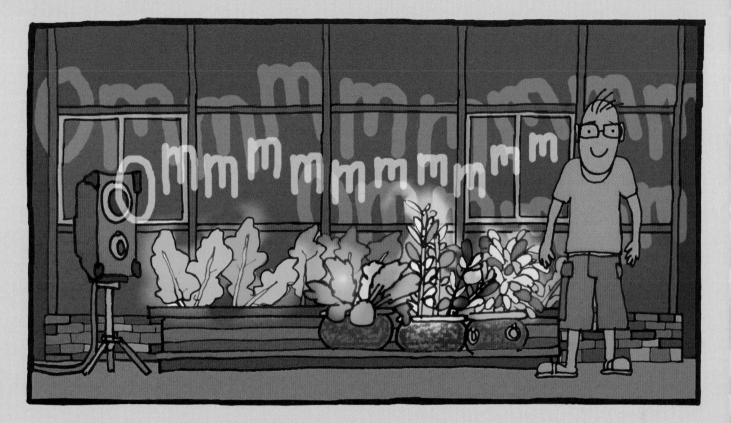

Grown within the frequency of the "OM" sound,
Graham's vegetables began to shine.

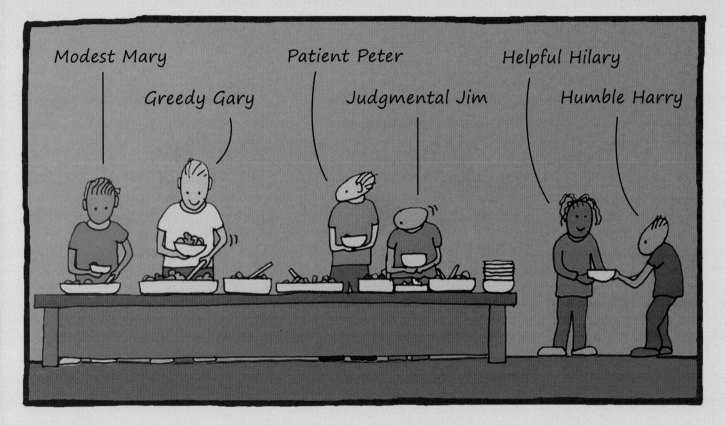

Mealtimes on meditation retreats.

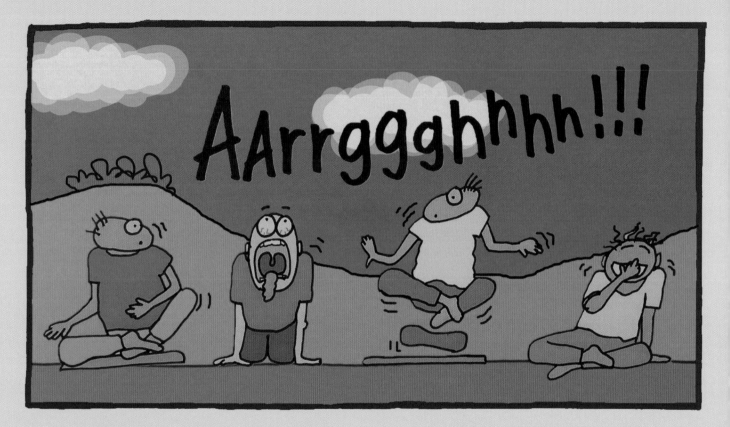

It was usually unsuspecting beginners that achieved spontaneous levitation during teacher Tom's epic demonstrations of the Lion's Roar technique.

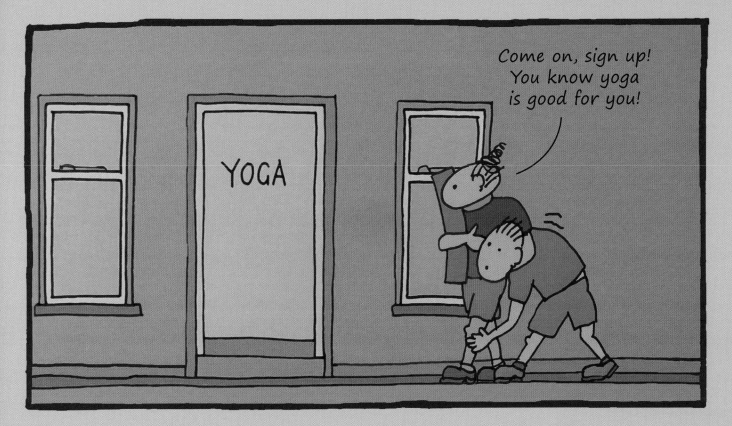

As competition increased,
the marketing tactics became more and more radical.

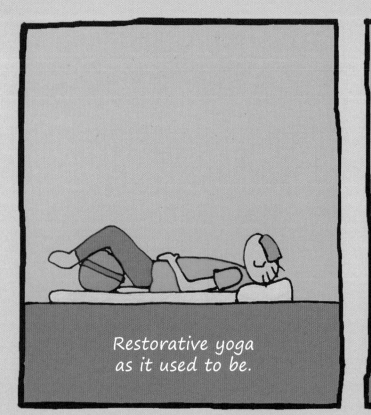

Restorative yoga
as it used to be.

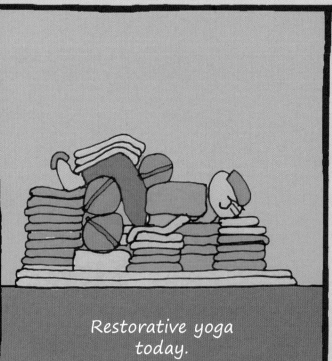

Restorative yoga
today.

John's meditation practice was giving rise to
some interesting philosophical contemplations.

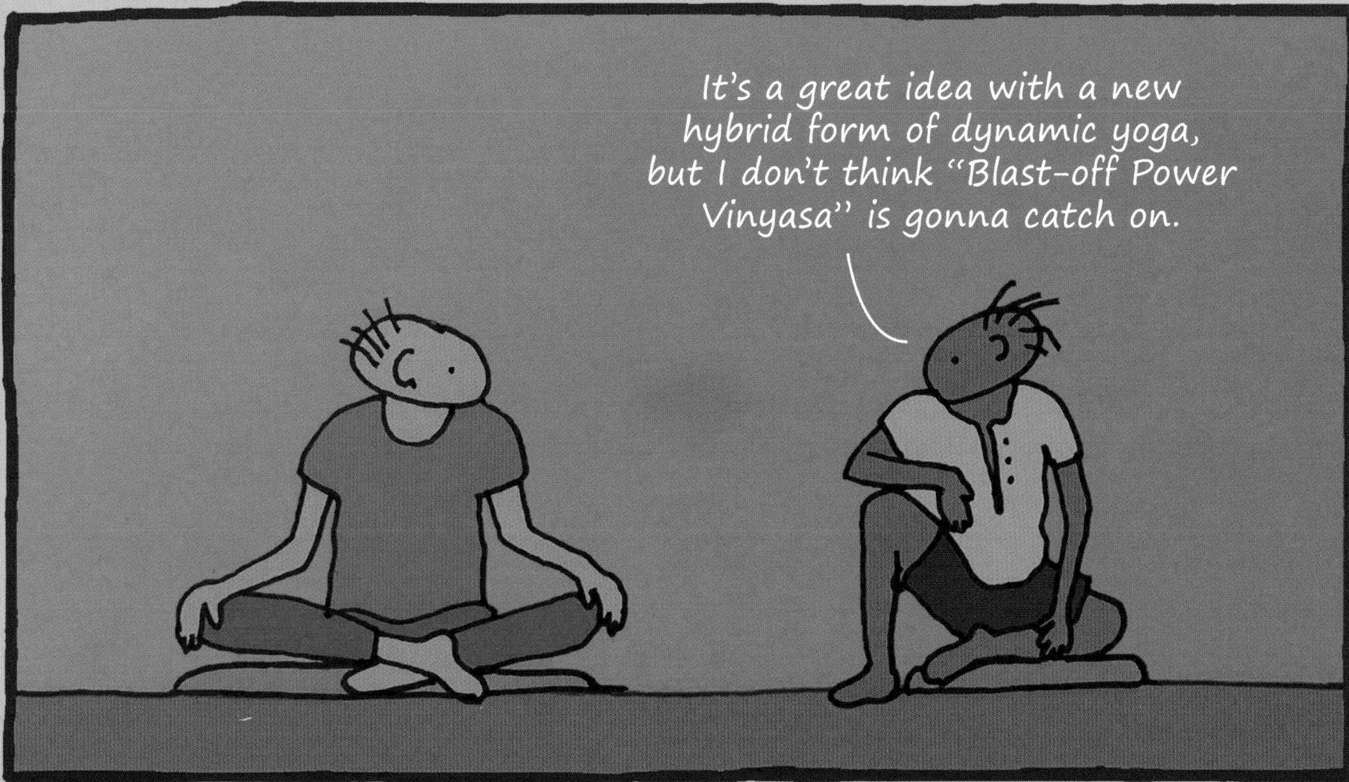
It's a great idea with a new hybrid form of dynamic yoga, but I don't think "Blast-off Power Vinyasa" is gonna catch on.

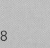

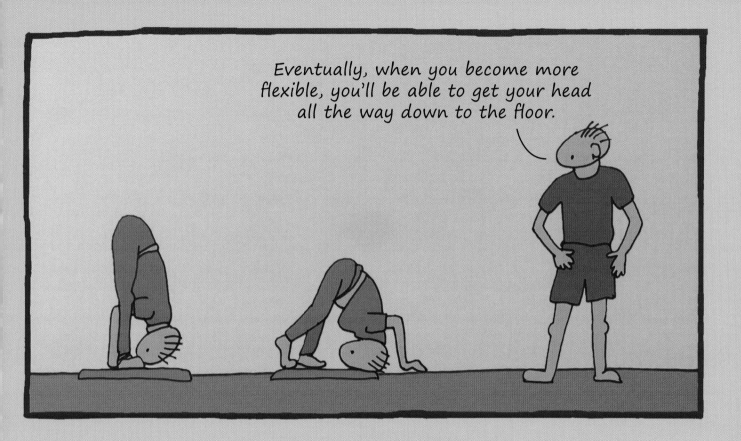

Why people need yoga teachers.

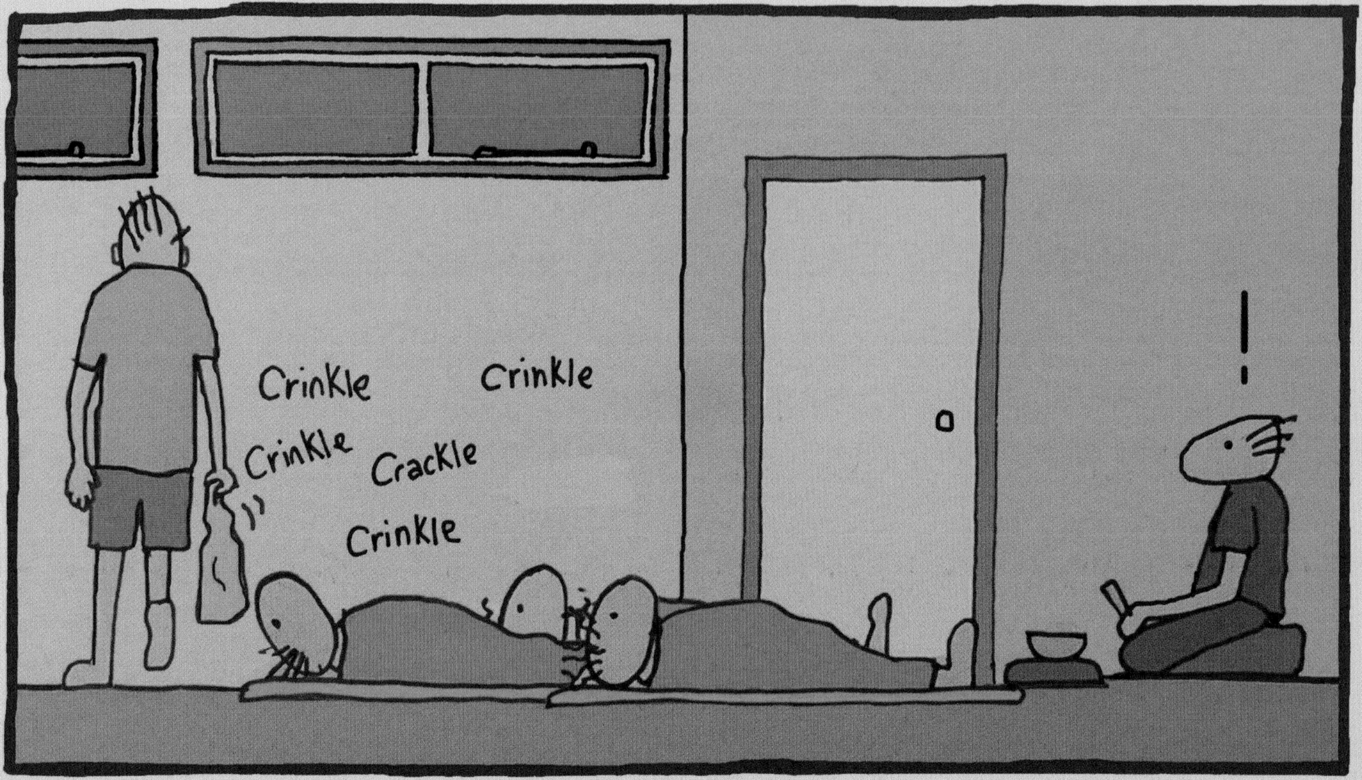
Crinkle
Crinkle
Crinkle
Crackle
Crinkle
!

George always left the class five minutes before the end of Savasana and seemed completely oblivious to the fact that he kept his stuff in the noisiest plastic bag on the planet.

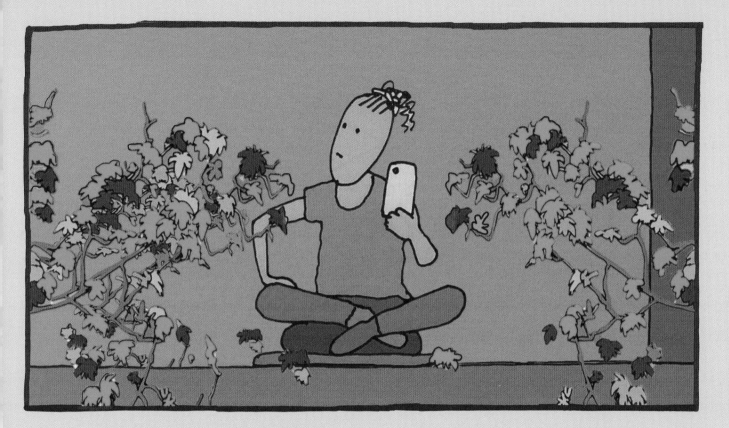

Mandy was on her eighth test shot and working hard to get that
"gazing into infinity" selfie for her next mindfulness event promo.

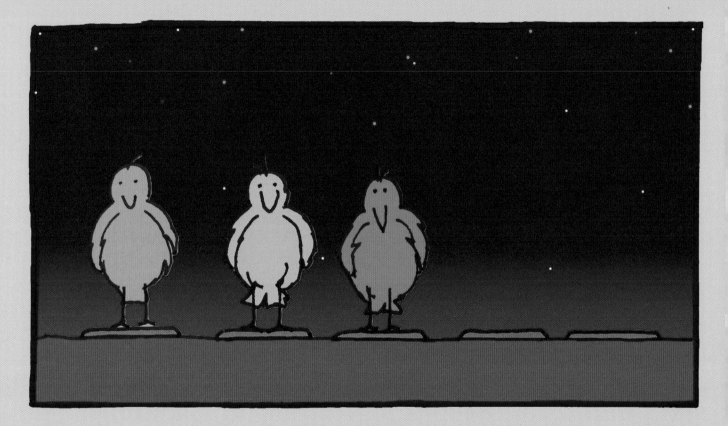

Despite the special Early Bird discounts,
there always seemed to be two spaces left.

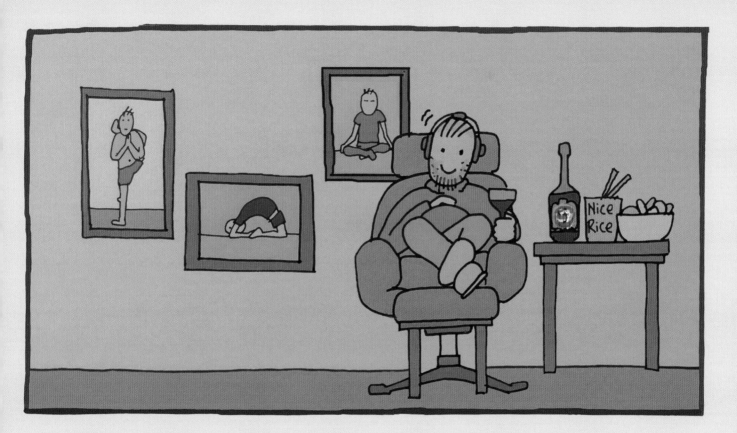

After 25 years of hardcore power yoga, Joe realized it was time to move beyond asana into higher levels of practice.

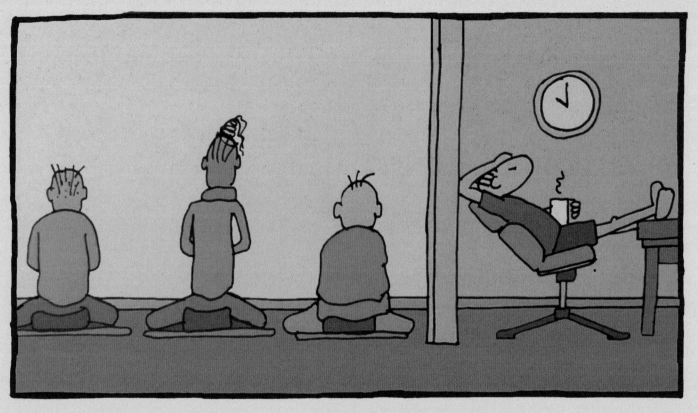

Teacher Steve had a bit of a banging hangover that morning, so he put the 10 a.m. students into a 45-minute White Wall meditation and then slipped into the next room for some chill and a coffee.

The Great Awakening was not happening
any time soon for Sandra.

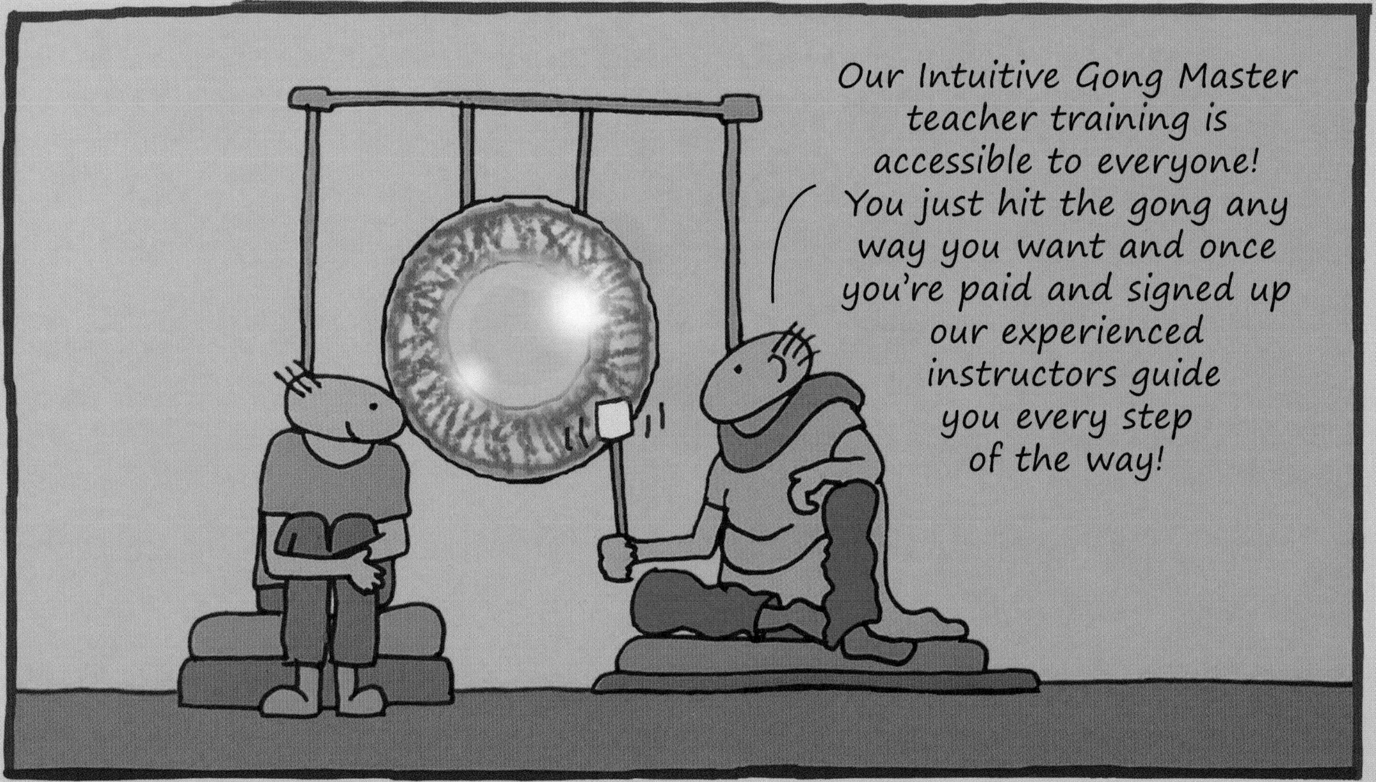
Our Intuitive Gong Master teacher training is accessible to everyone! You just hit the gong any way you want and once you're paid and signed up our experienced instructors guide you every step of the way!

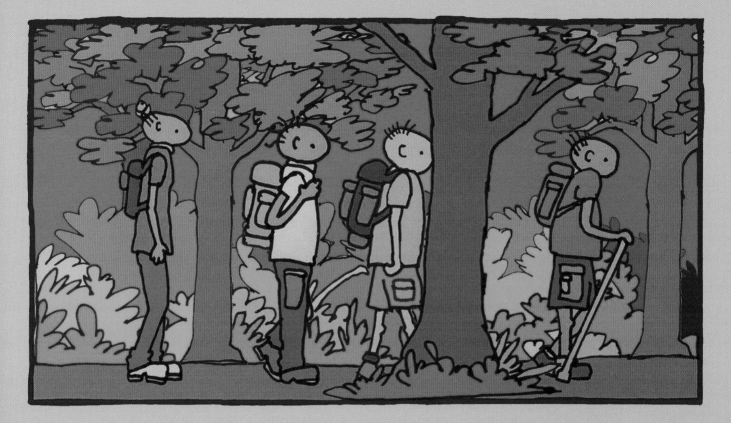

It slowly dawned on the "Mindfulness in the forest" participants
that they had actually paid to go for a walk in the woods.

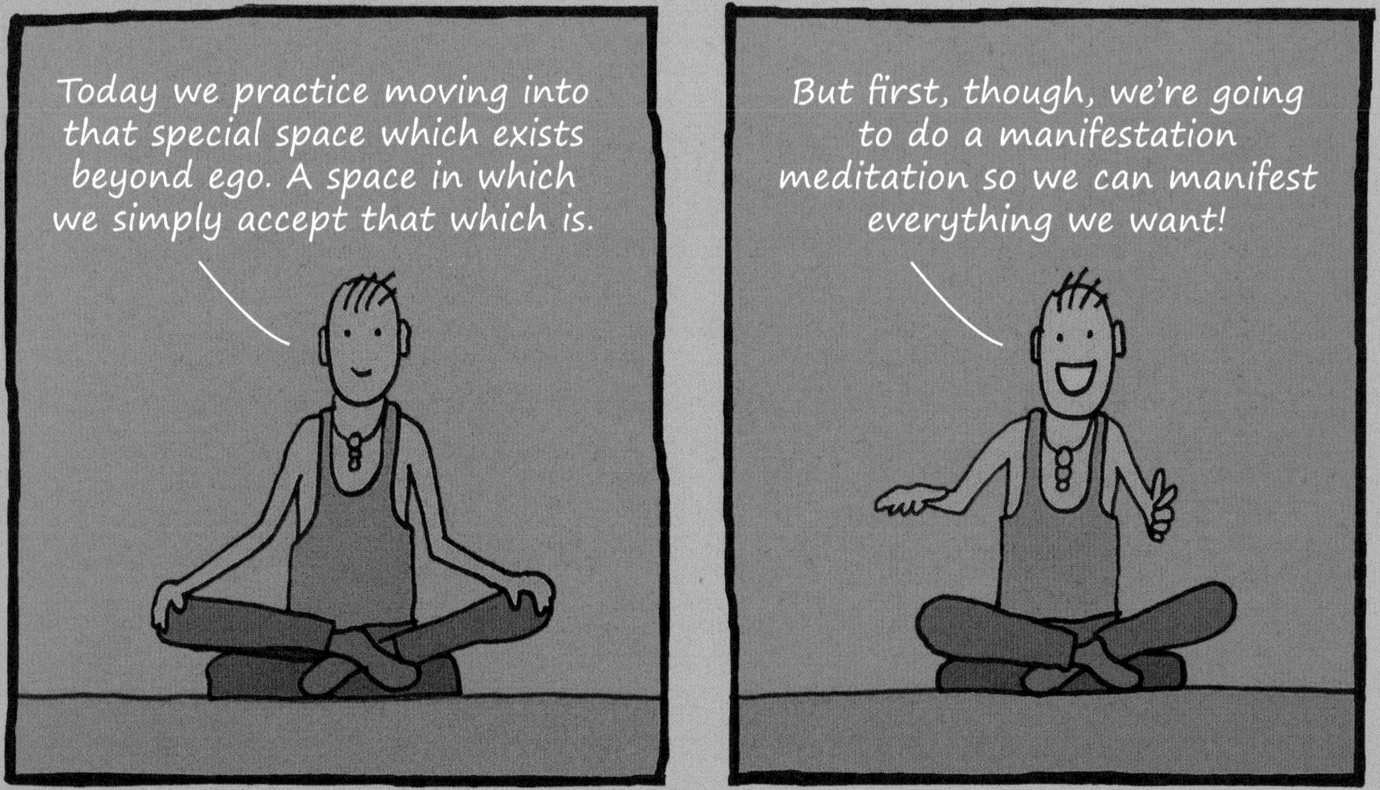
Today we practice moving into that special space which exists beyond ego. A space in which we simply accept that which is.
But first, though, we're going to do a manifestation meditation so we can manifest everything we want!

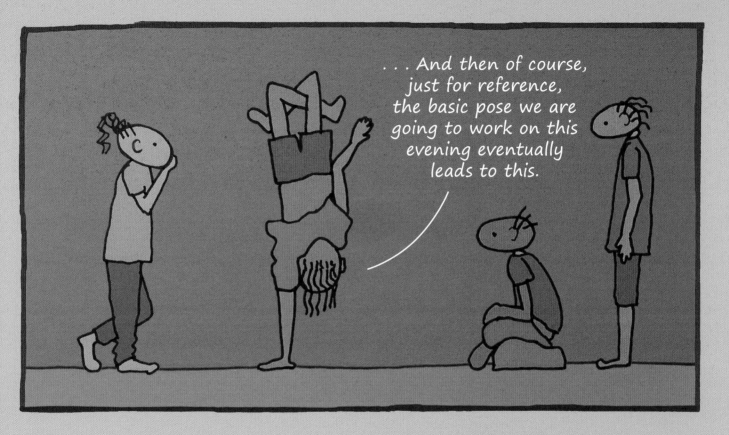

When advanced yoga teachers just can't help showing off.

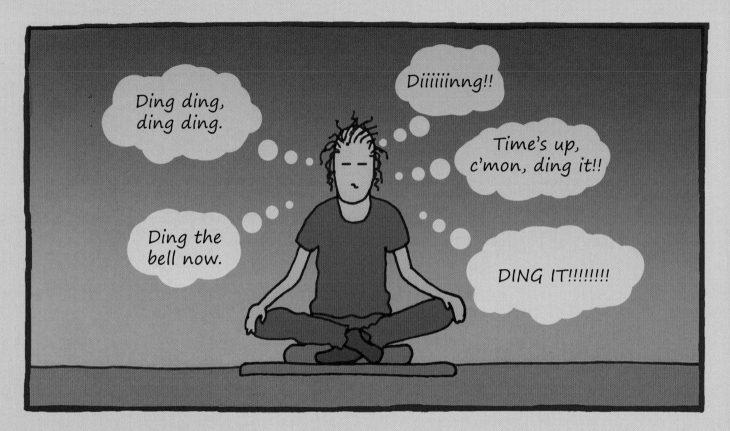

Martin was a beginner to meditation and as usual, toward the end of the 45-minute meditation, all traces of virtue were fading rapidly.

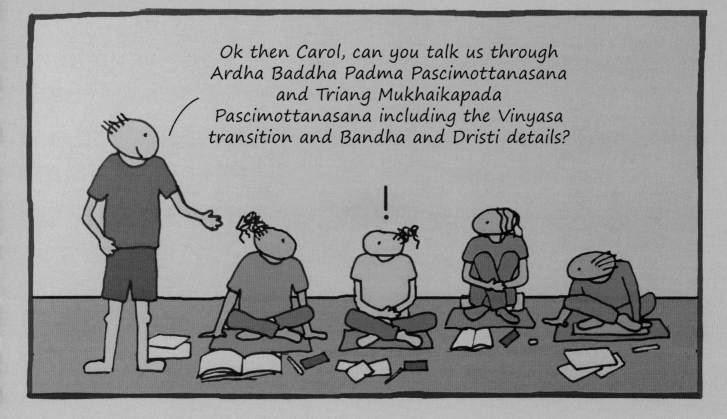

When the 500-hour teacher trainees find out
they are not as advanced as they thought they were.

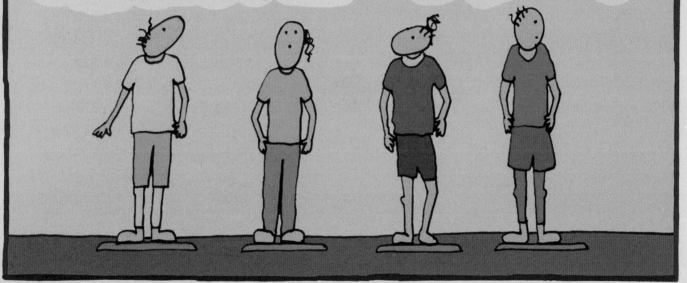

Inspired by the Urban Retreat theme of "traveling without moving,"
teacher Dan experimented with a new theme of "teaching without being there."

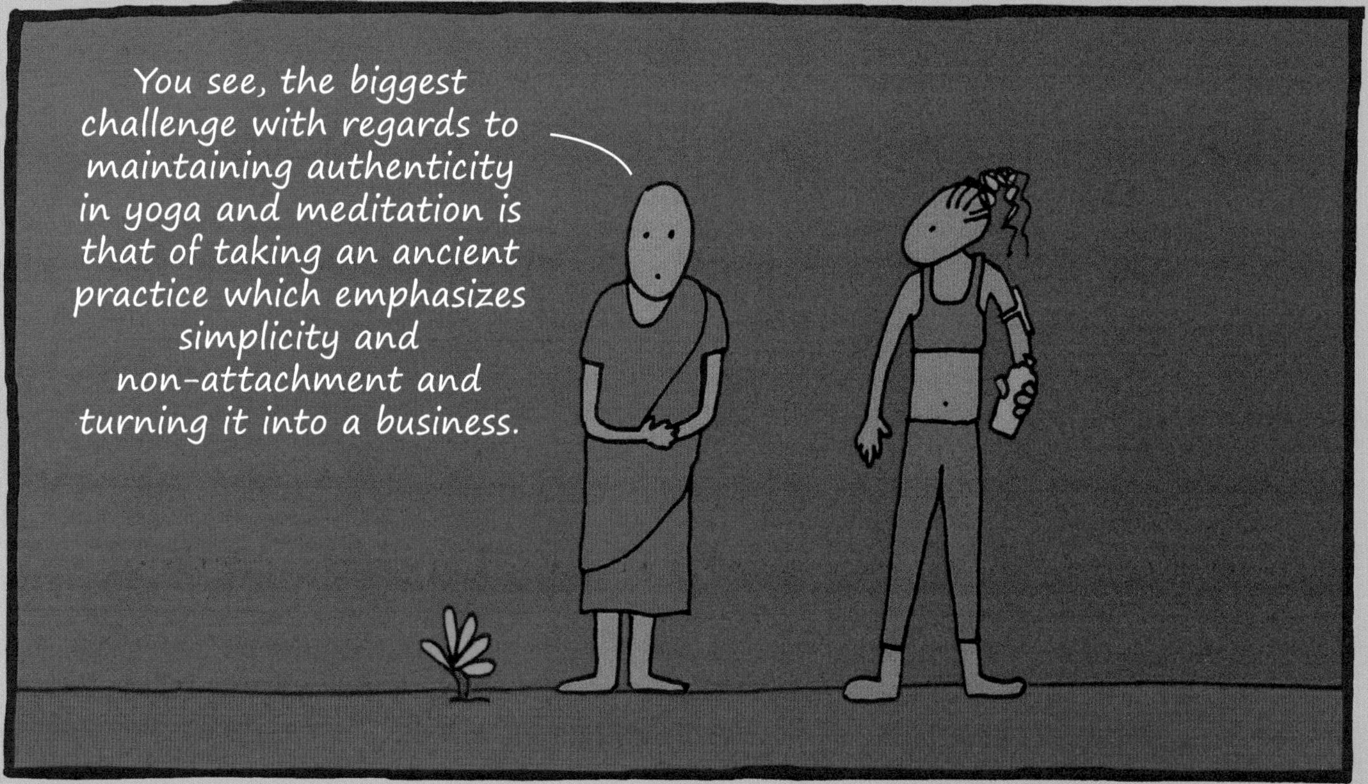
You see, the biggest challenge with regards to maintaining authenticity in yoga and meditation is that of taking an ancient practice which emphasizes simplicity and non-attachment and turning it into a business.

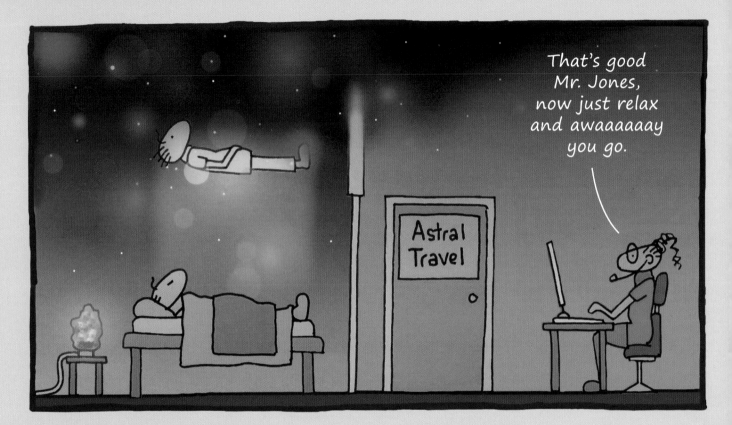

Many tour companies were struggling in the Corona crisis,
but for Astral Travel, business was booming.

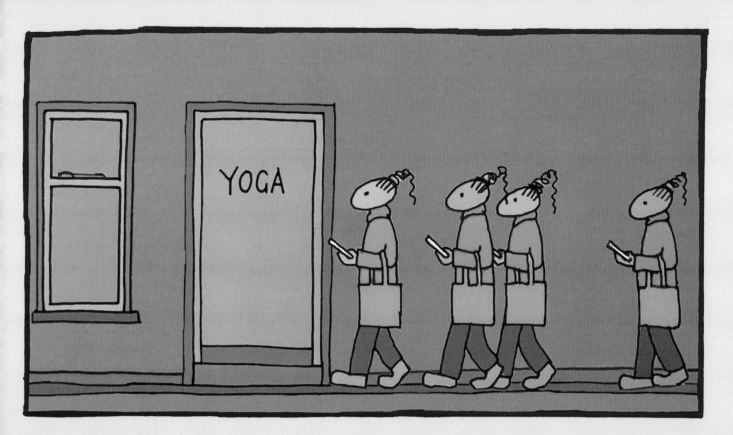

The participants began to arrive for the "You are unique" workshop.

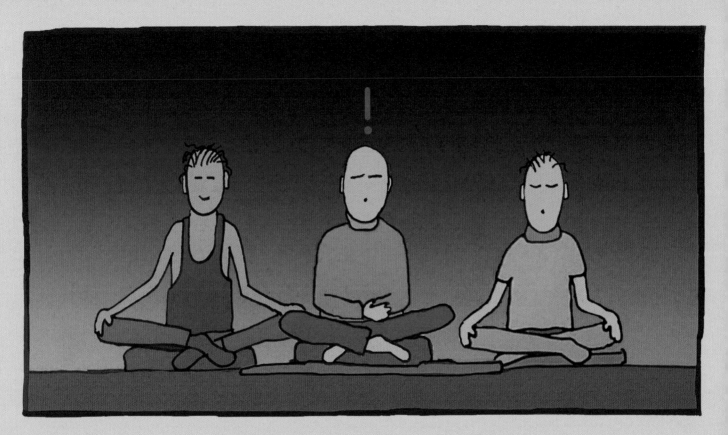

After 45 minutes of sitting meditation, Simon wasn't sure if he was levitating or whether his ass had just gone numb.

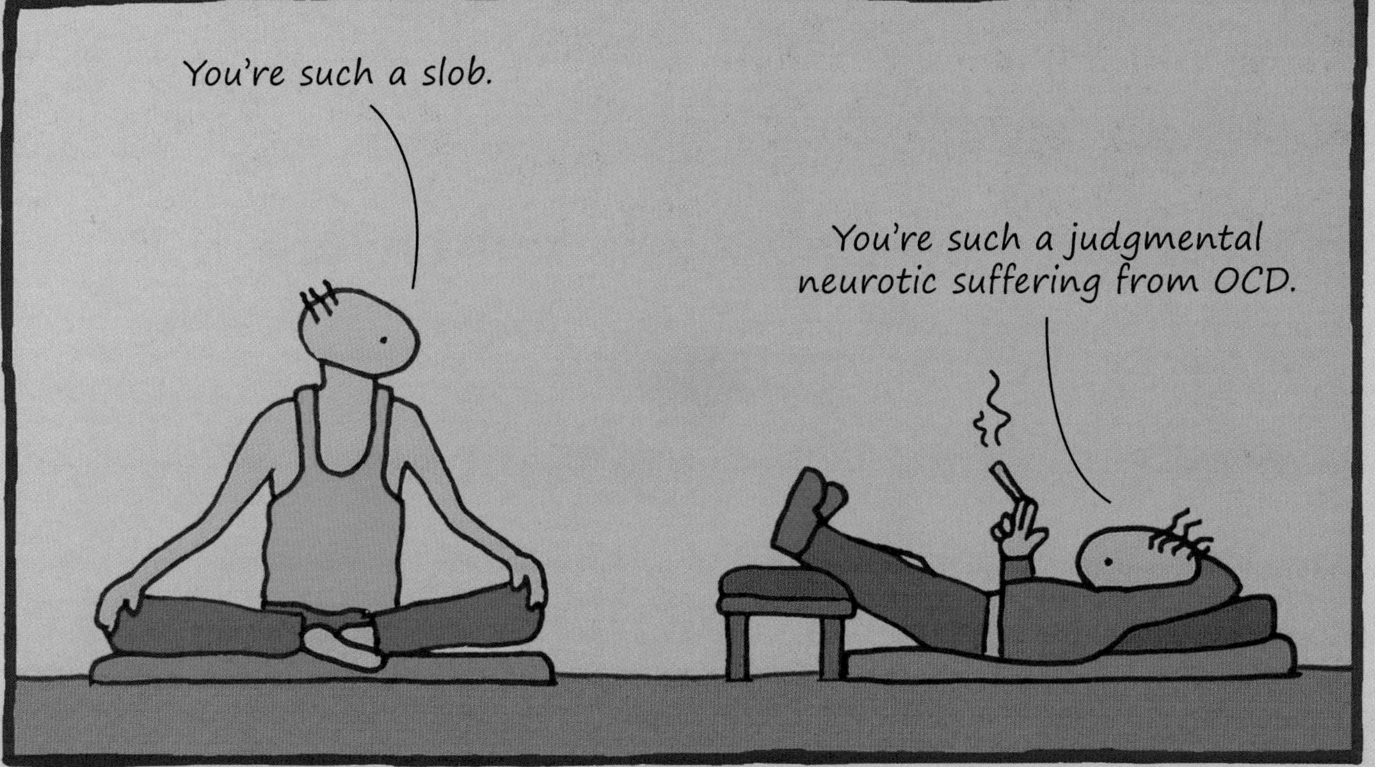

You're such a slob.
You're such a judgmental neurotic suffering from OCD.

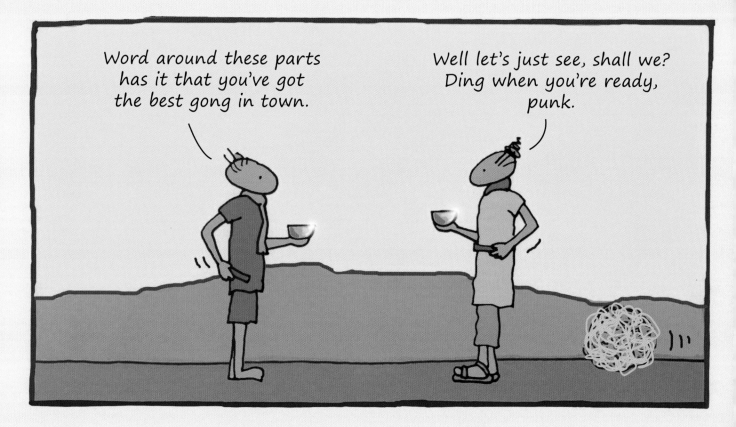

Gong fight at the OK Corral.

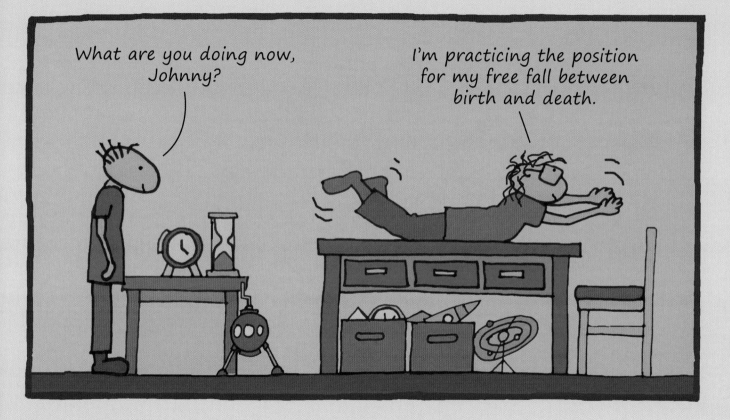

For Cosmic Johnny,
there were no ordinary moments.

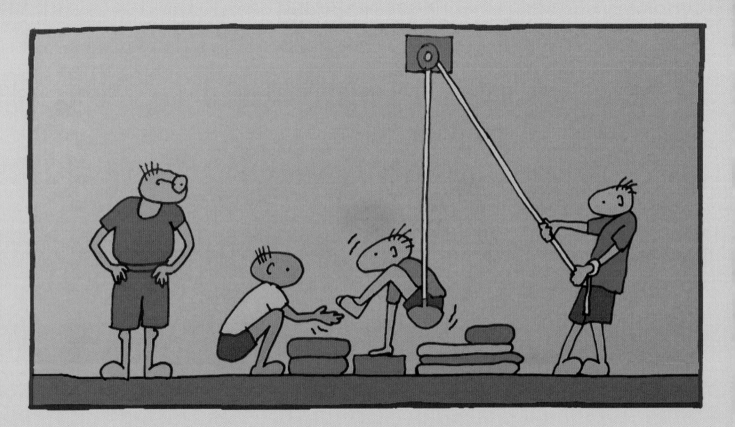

Teacher Brian was satisfied that all the safety requirements
were being adhered to during the Arm-balance Intensive workshop.

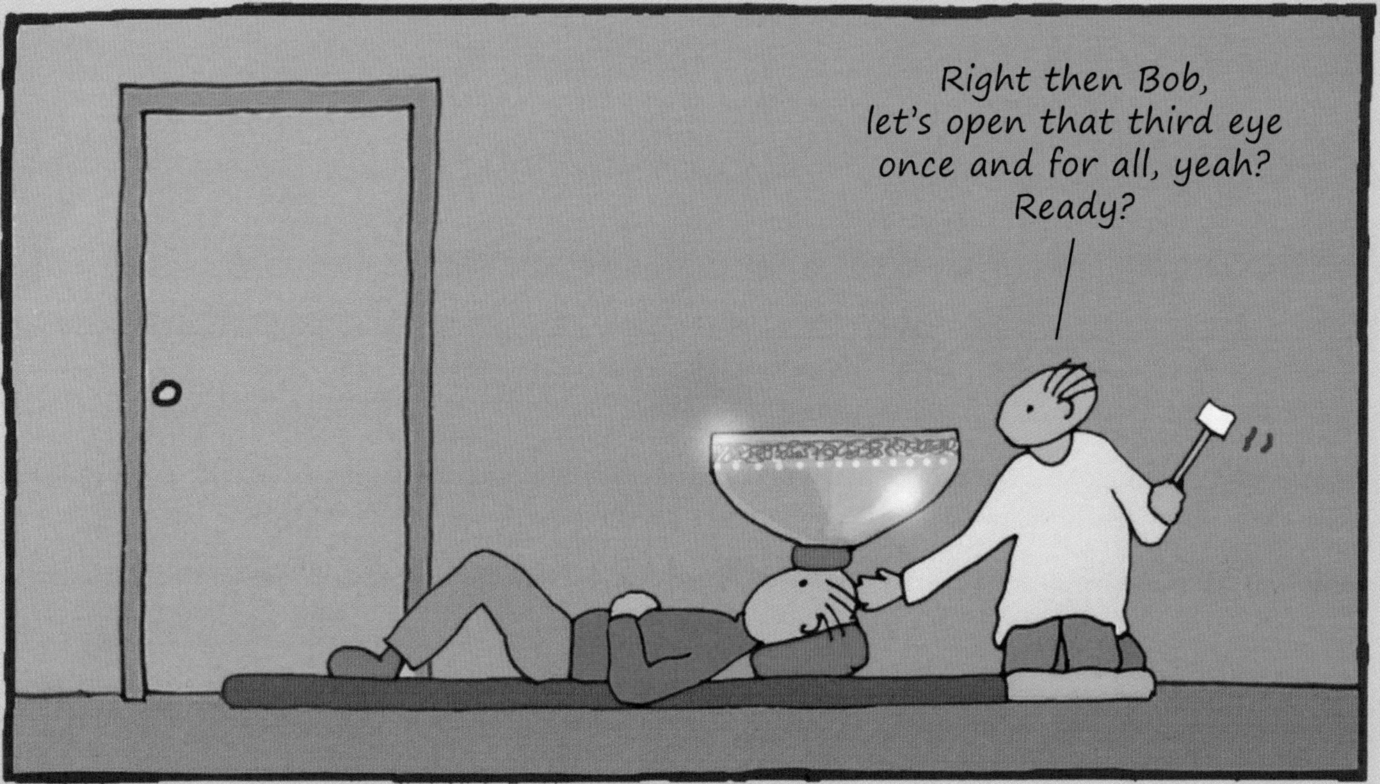
Right then Bob,
let's open that third eye
once and for all, yeah?
Ready?

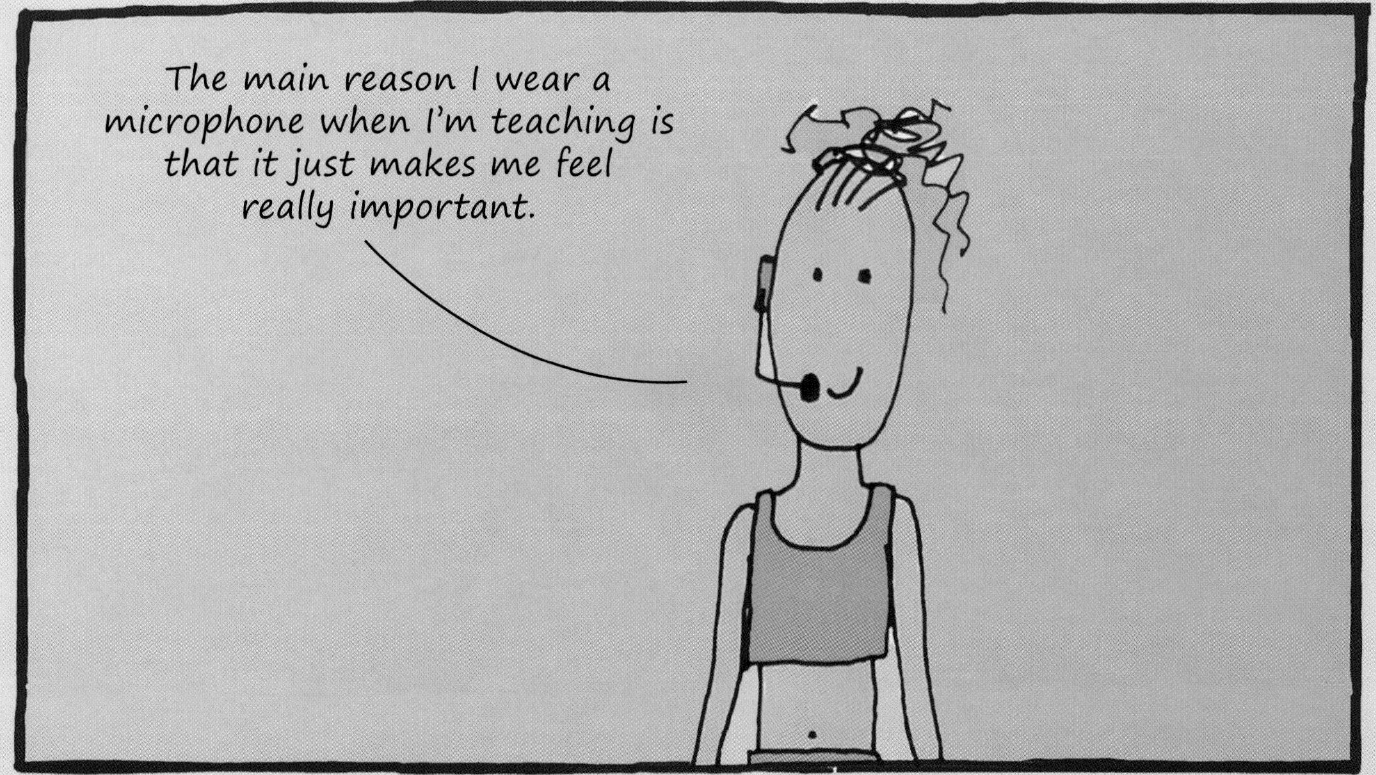
The main reason I wear a microphone when I'm teaching is that it just makes me feel really important.

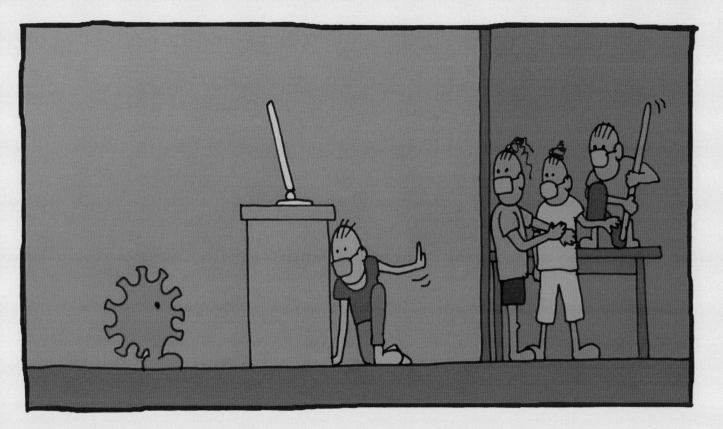

Everyone took defense position protocol when Corona came in
to sign up for the Pranayama Intensive.

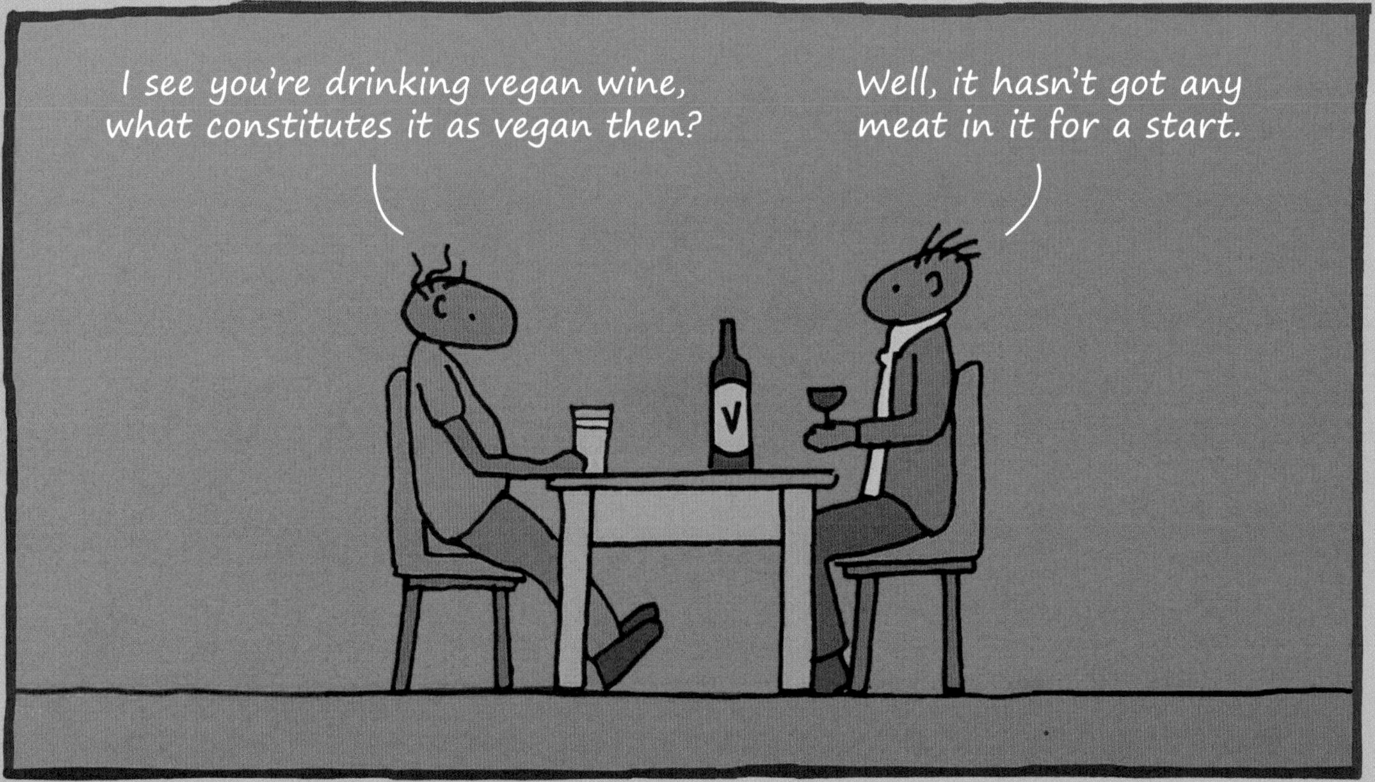
I see you're drinking vegan wine, what constitutes it as vegan then?
Well, it hasn't got any meat in it for a start.
V

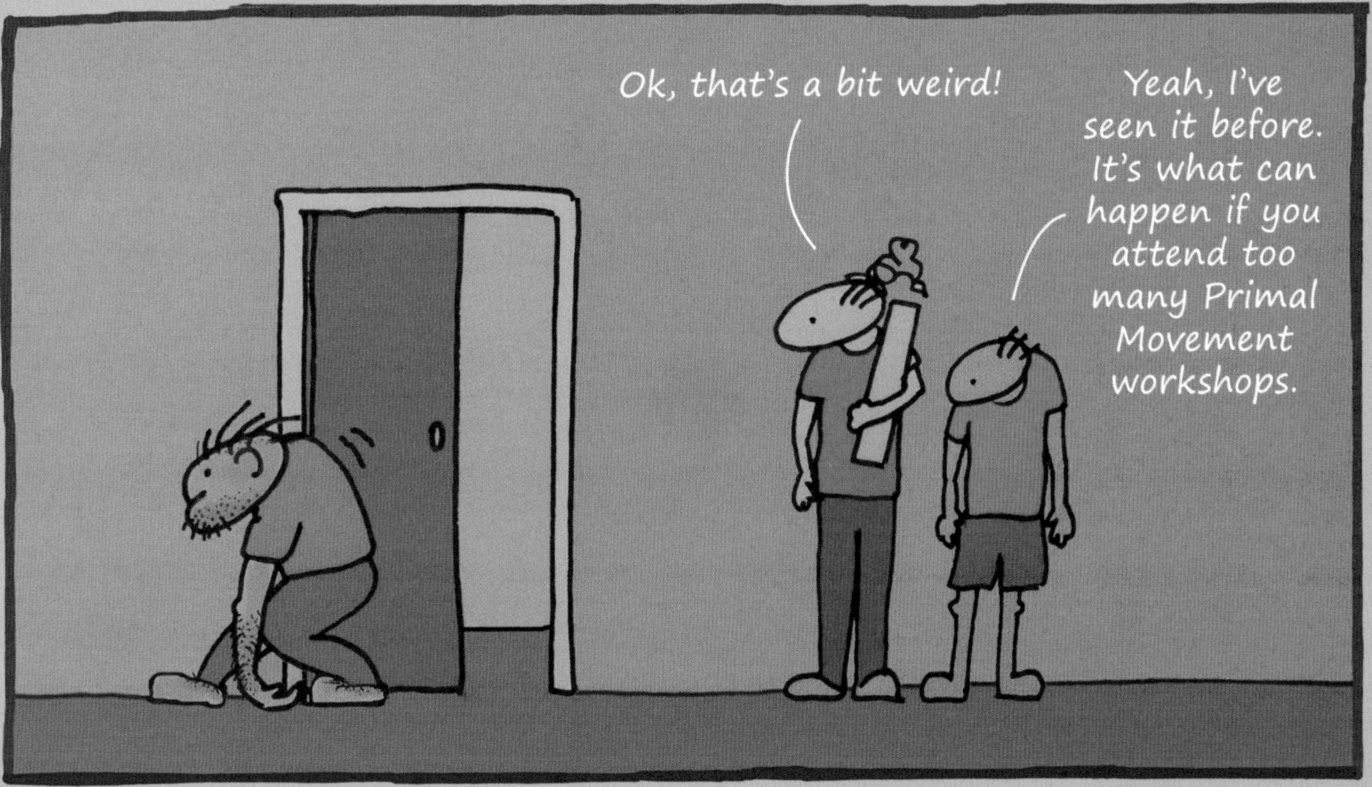

Ok, that's a bit weird!
Yeah, I've seen it before. It's what can happen if you attend too many Primal Movement workshops.

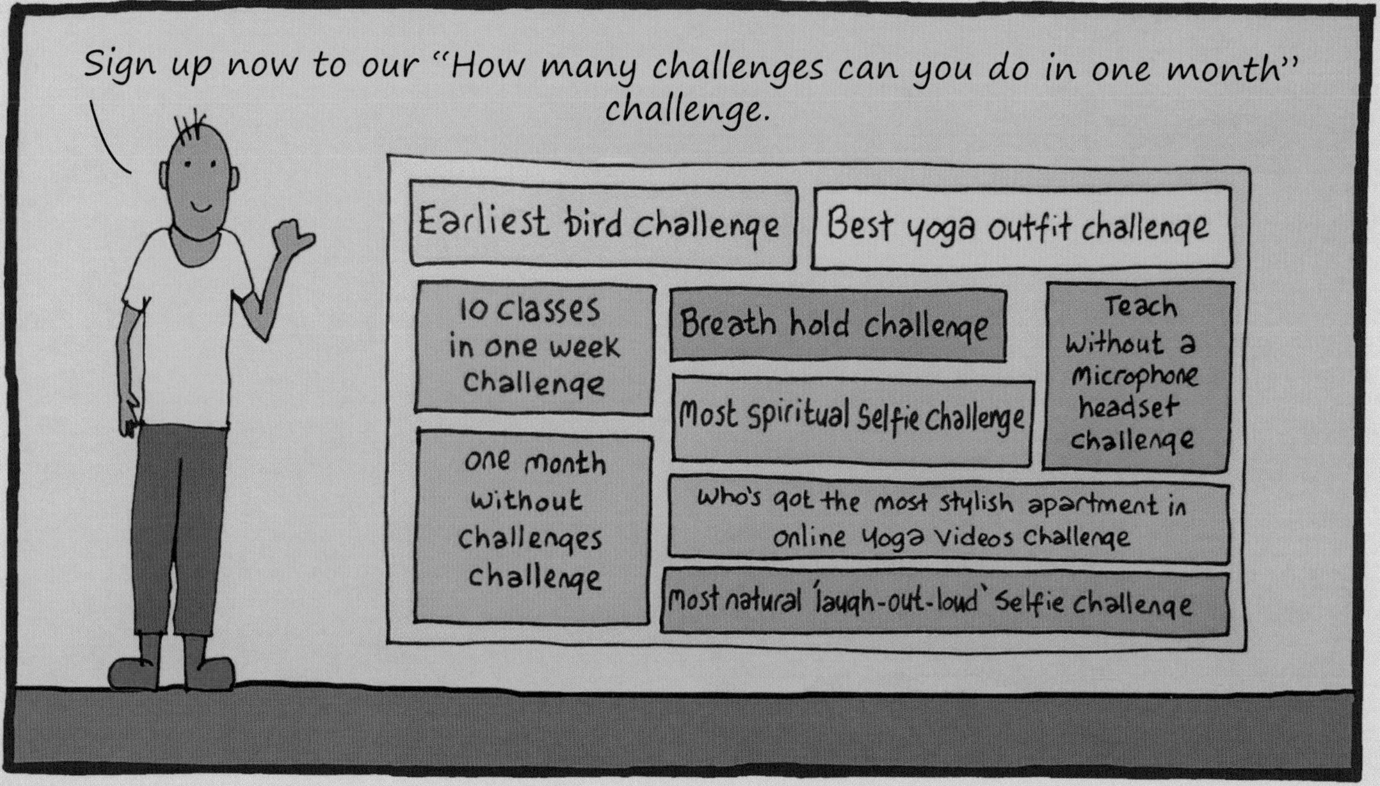
Sign up now to our "How many challenges can you do in one month" challenge.
Earliest bird challenge
Best yoga outfit challenge
10 classes in one week challenge
Breath hold challenge
Teach without a microphone headset challenge
Most spiritual selfie challenge
one month without challenges challenge
Who's got the most stylish apartment in online yoga videos challenge
Most natural 'laugh-out-loud' selfie challenge

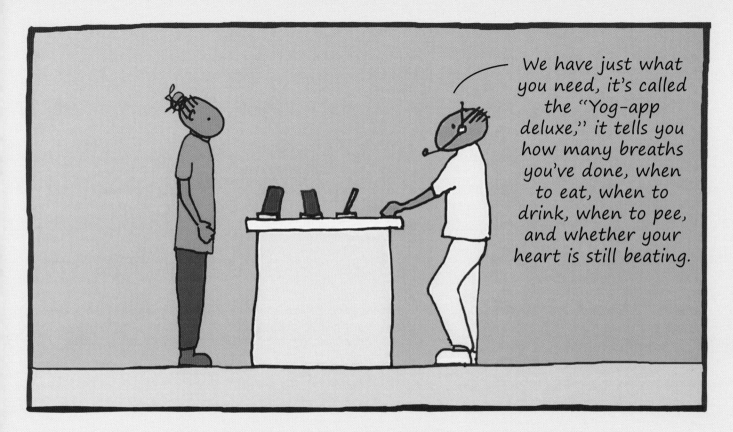

The Yog-app deluxe, guaranteed to remove all natural intuition over a three month period or your money back.

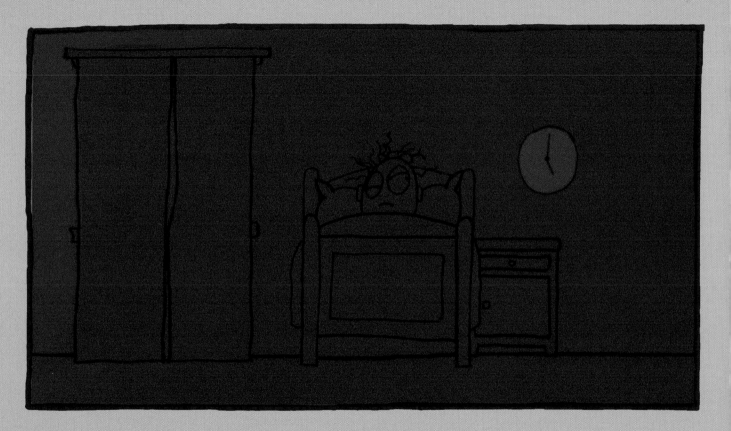

Emily was really beginning to feel all the benefits
of the 10-day early morning Vinyasa Intensive Challenge.

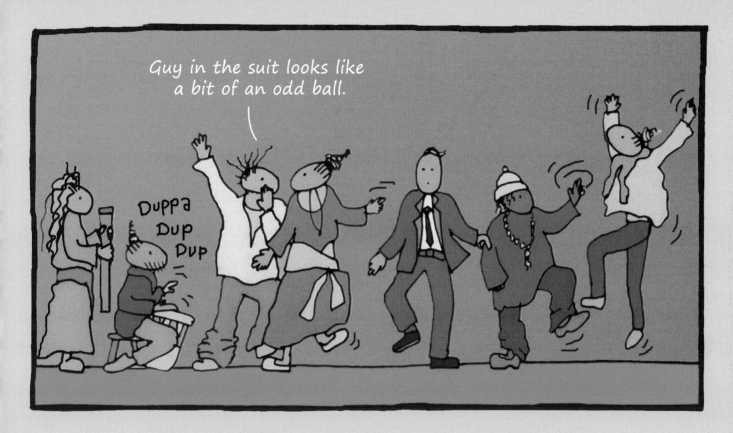

John decided to try out a bit of self-expression
at the monthly Spiritual Dance Festival.

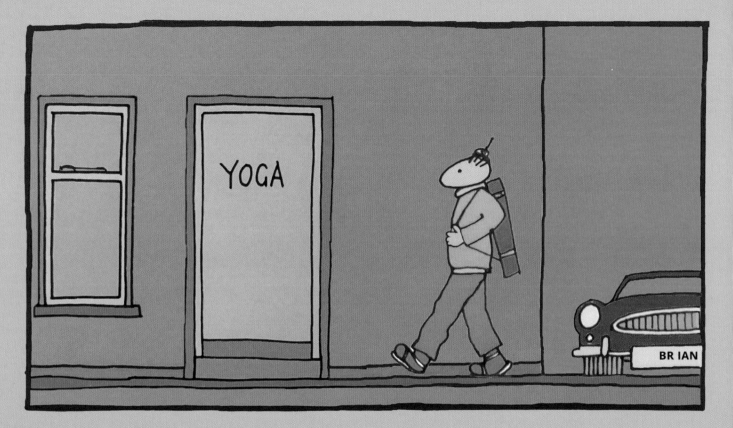

For millionaire Brian, teaching yoga wasn't about the money,
for him it was a calling, a passion.

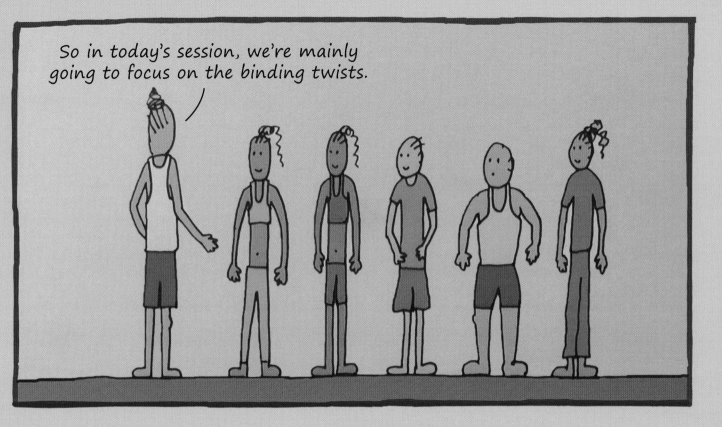

Another challenging session for Bob.

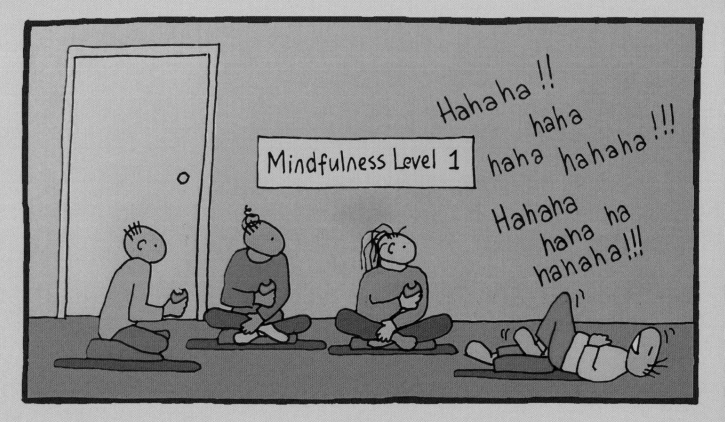

After five minutes of slow-motion silent apple eating,
Jim just couldn't contain it any longer.

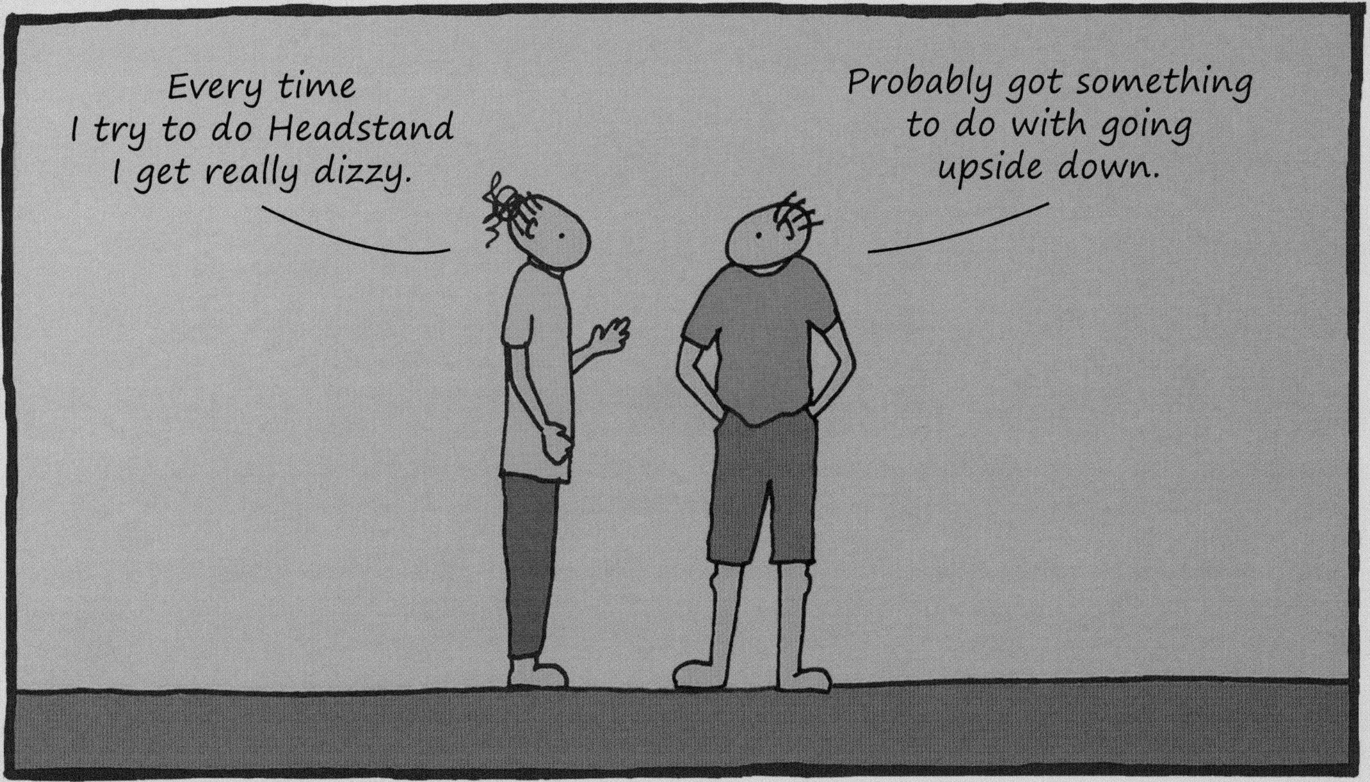
Every time
I try to do Headstand
I get really dizzy.
Probably got something
to do with going
upside down.

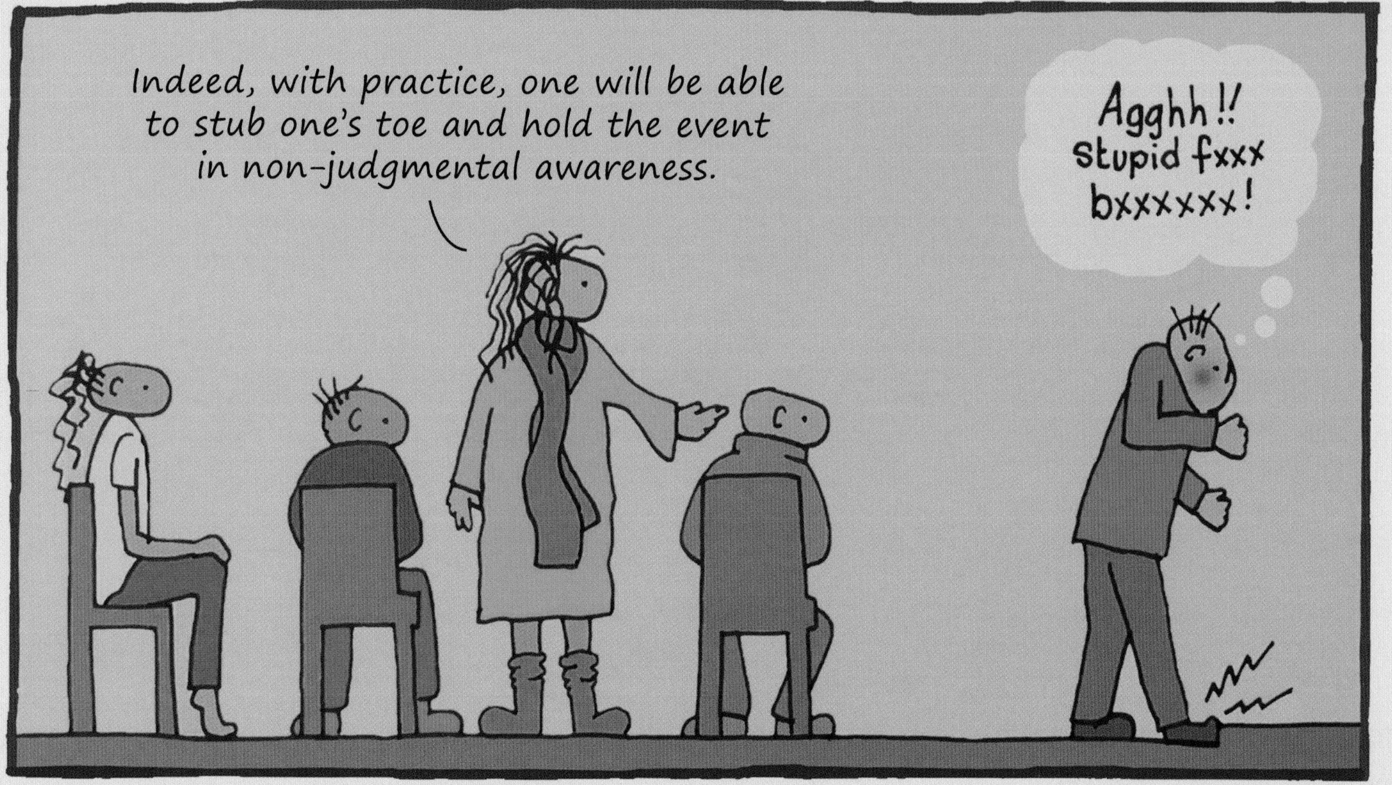
Indeed, with practice, one will be able to stub one's toe and hold the event in non-judgmental awareness.
Agghh!! stupid fxxx bxxxxxx!

Mindfulness Level 2.

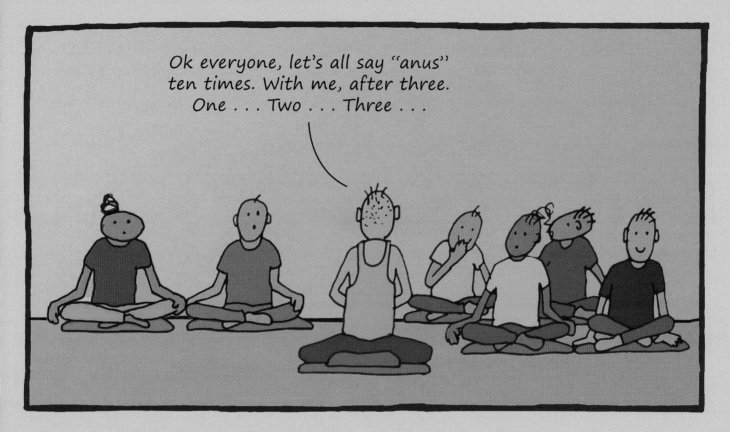

Teacher Jack decided to get everyone comfortable with the main element of the Mula Bandha workshop right from the start.

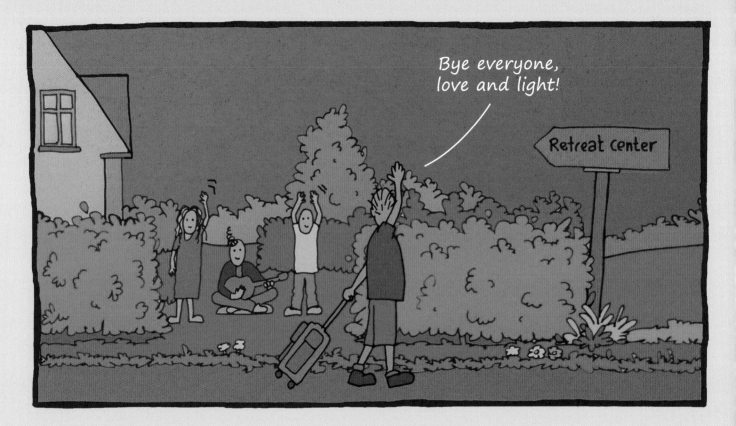

After a week of hugs, smiles, and inner bliss, Derek couldn't wait
to get to that pepperoni pizza, six-pack of booze, and the adult channel.

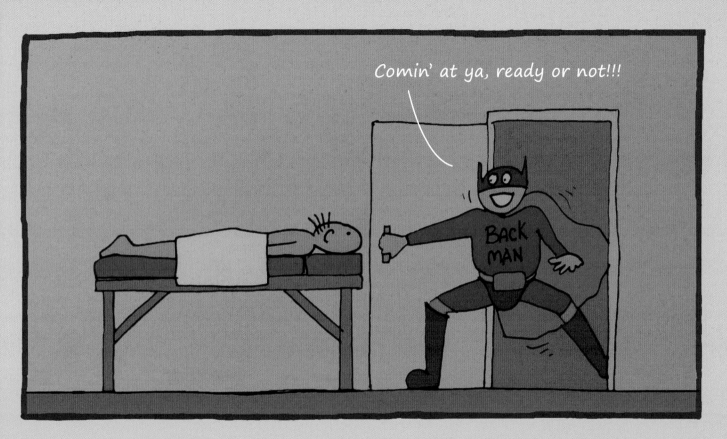

The brochure promised a radical new approach guaranteed
to take your mind off your back problems.

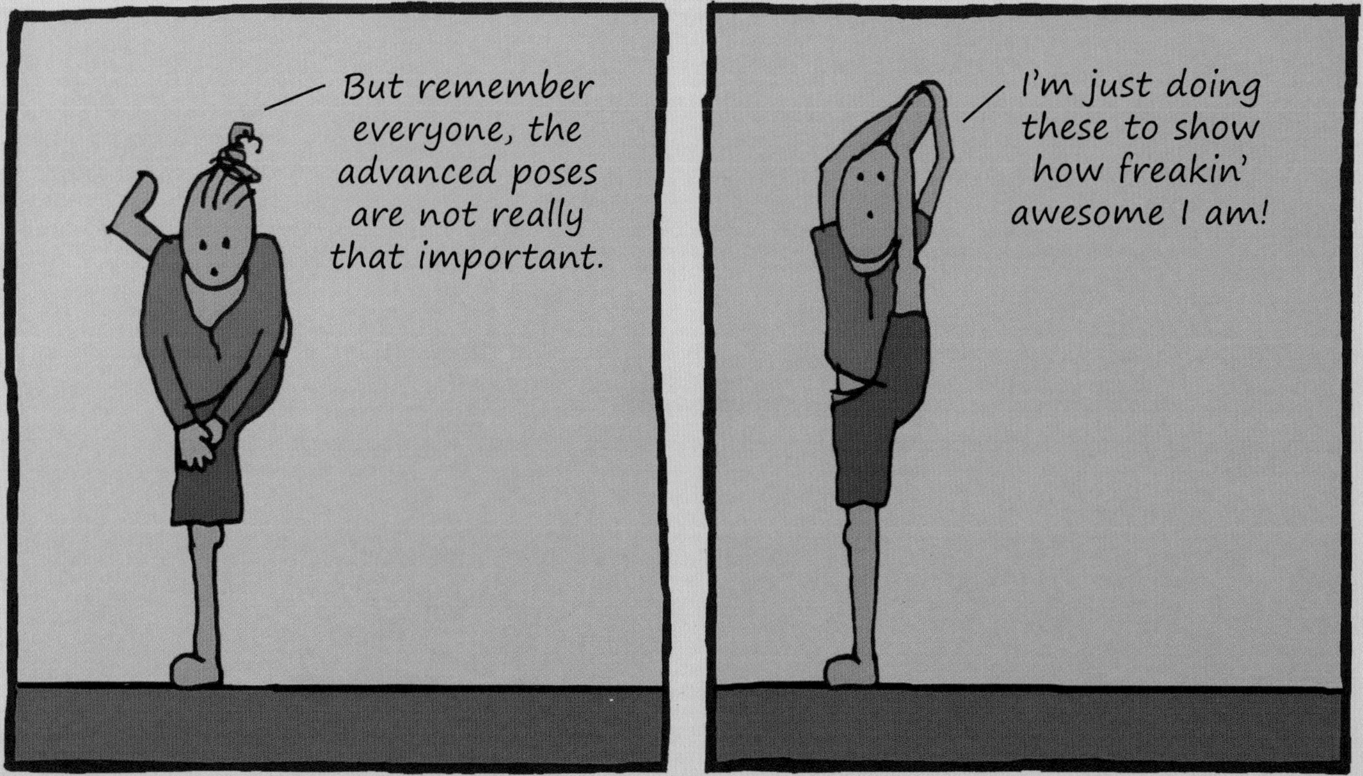
But remember everyone, the advanced poses are not really that important.
I'm just doing these to show how freakin' awesome I am!

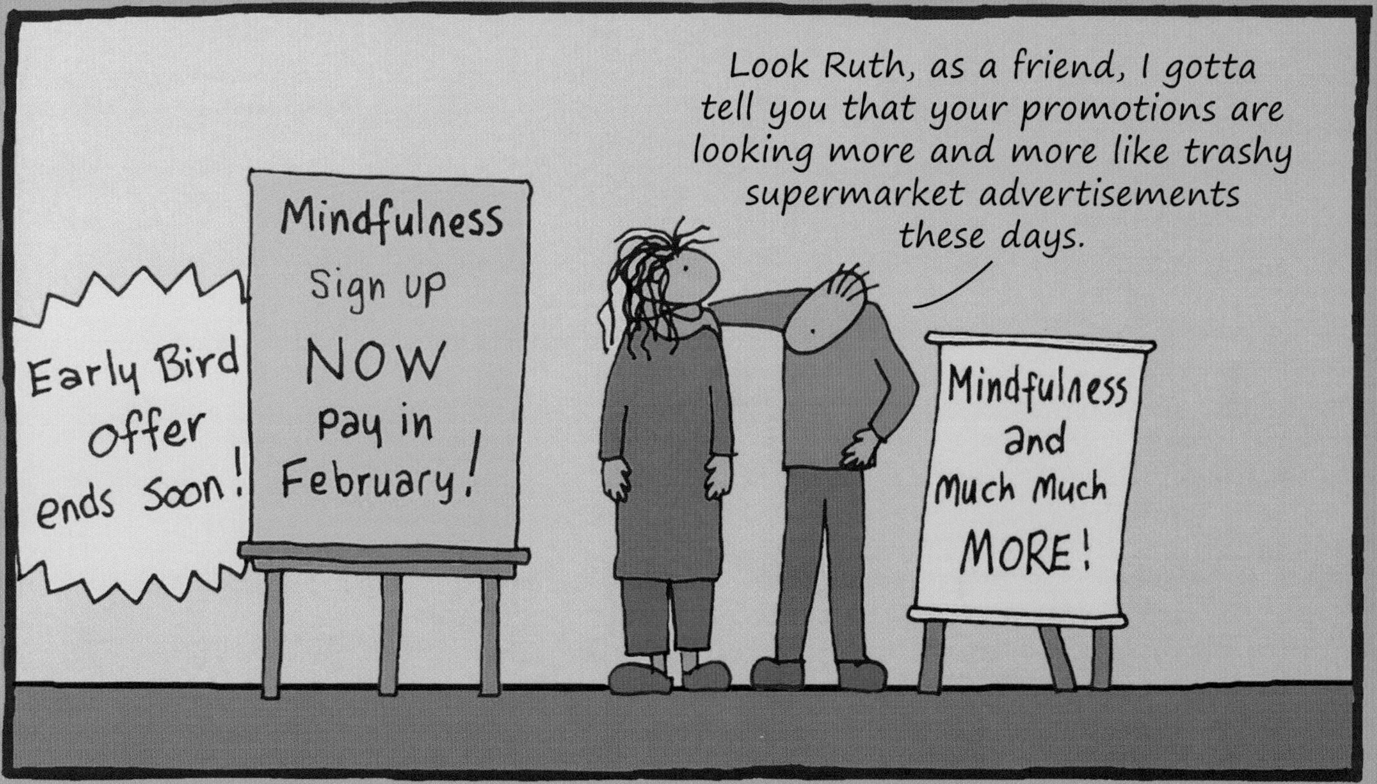

Look Ruth, as a friend, I gotta tell you that your promotions are looking more and more like trashy supermarket advertisements these days.
Early Bird offer ends soon!
Mindfulness Sign up NOW pay in February!
Mindfulness and much much MORE!

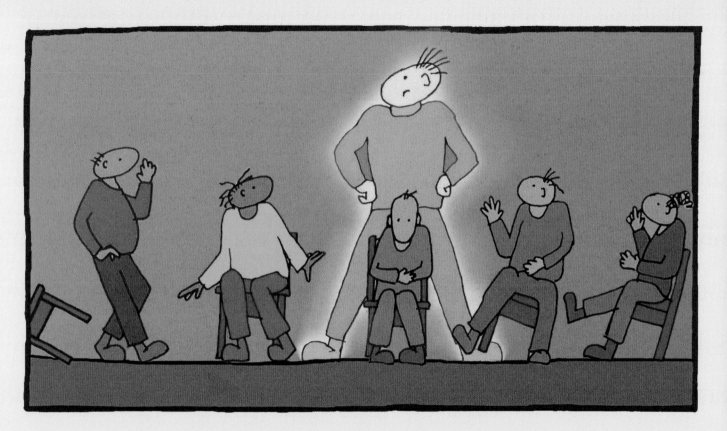

During the meditation discussion,
Humble Harry's ego suddenly manifested behind him.

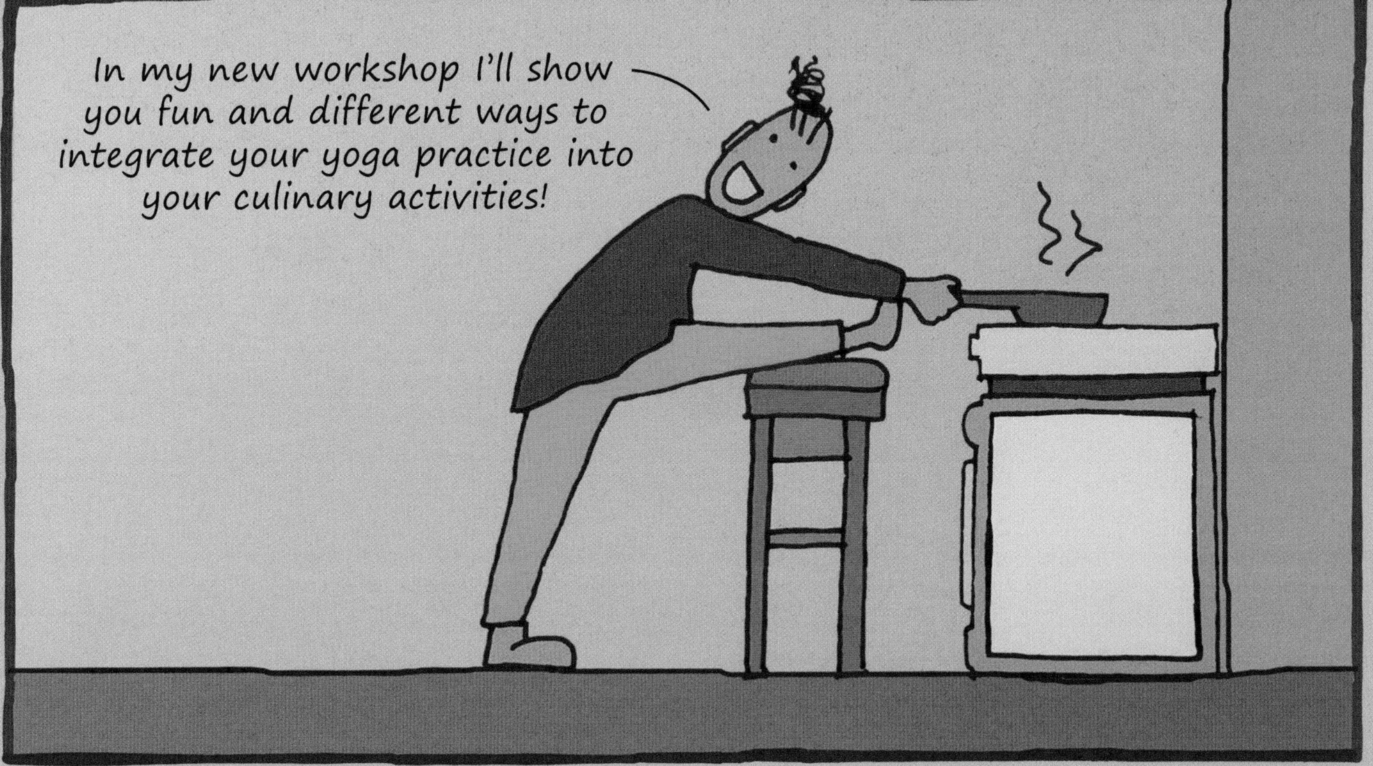
In my new workshop I'll show you fun and different ways to integrate your yoga practice into your culinary activities!

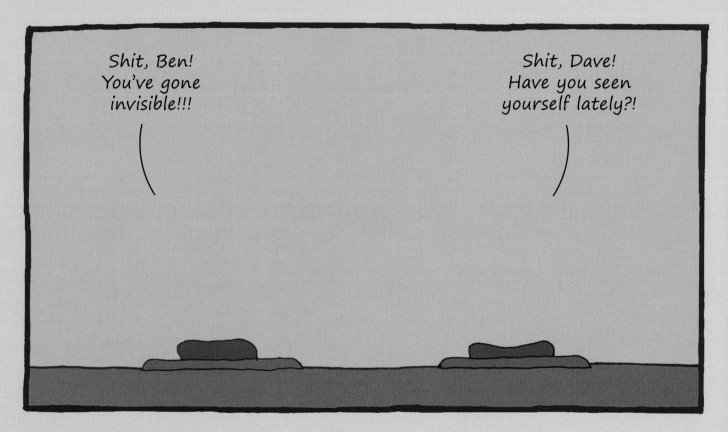

When pranayama students overdo it.

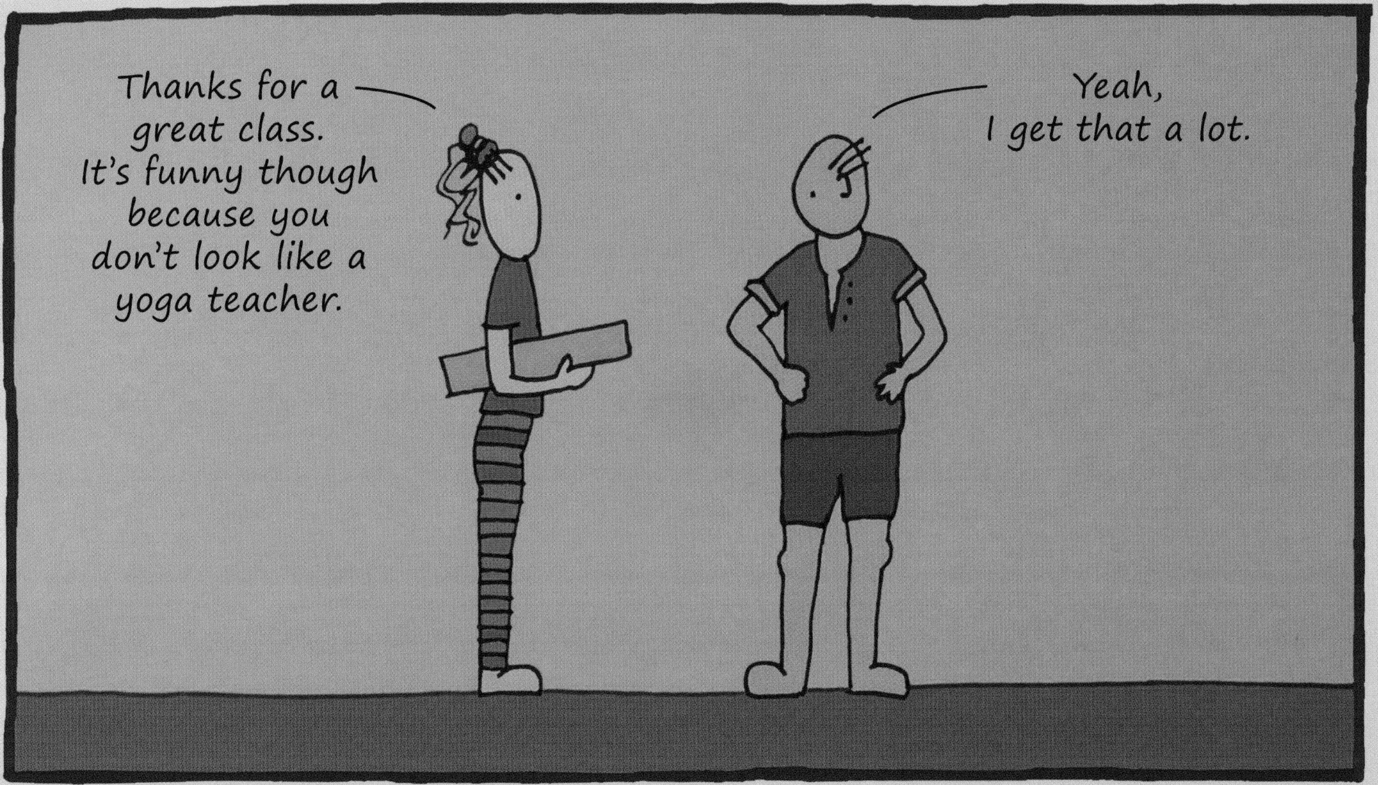
Thanks for a great class. It's funny though because you don't look like a yoga teacher.
Yeah, I get that a lot.

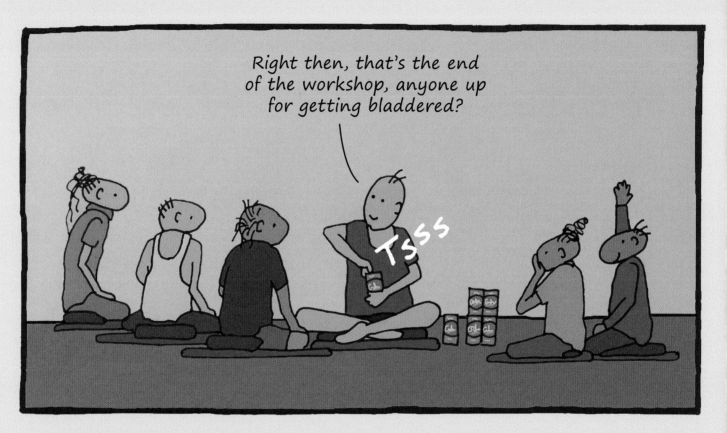

Teacher Dan had a very effective way of
preventing students from putting him on a pedestal.

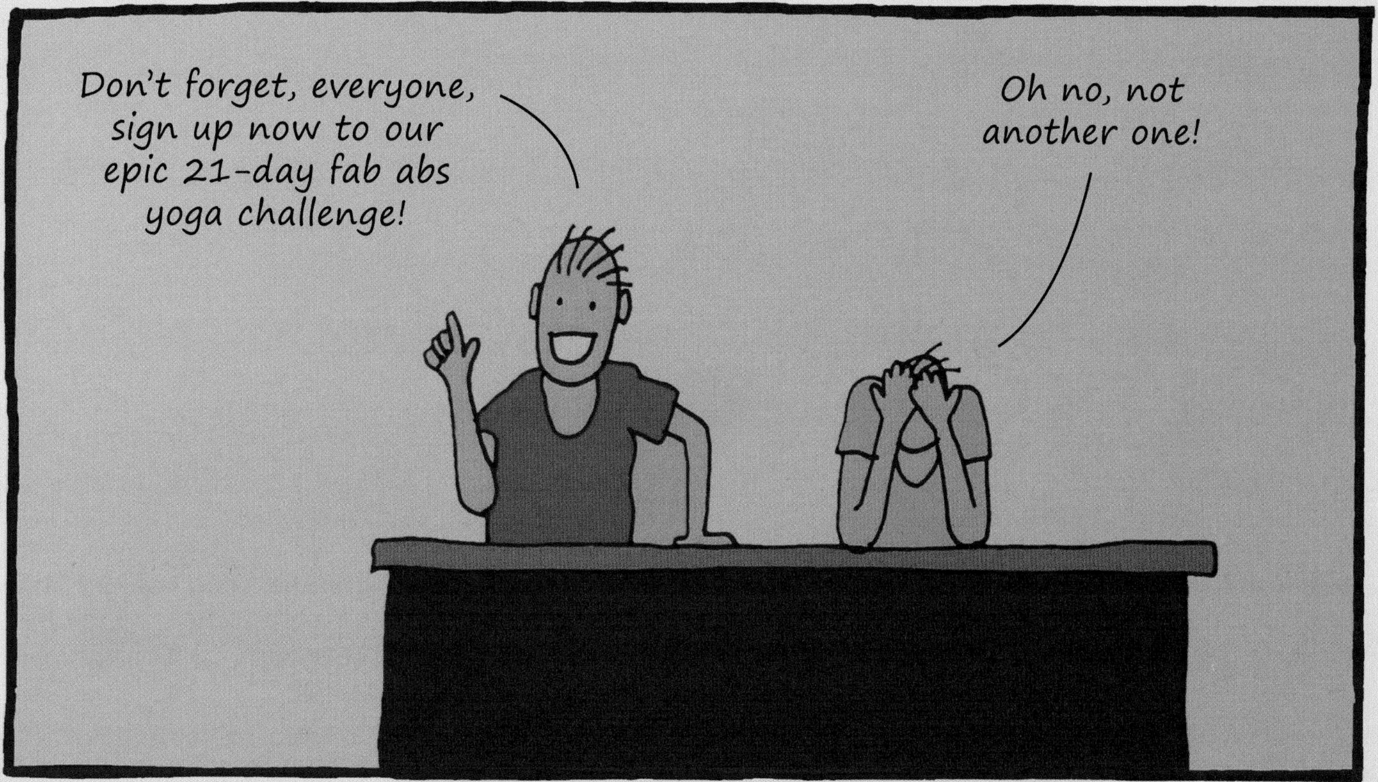
Don't forget, everyone, sign up now to our epic 21-day fab abs yoga challenge!
Oh no, not another one!

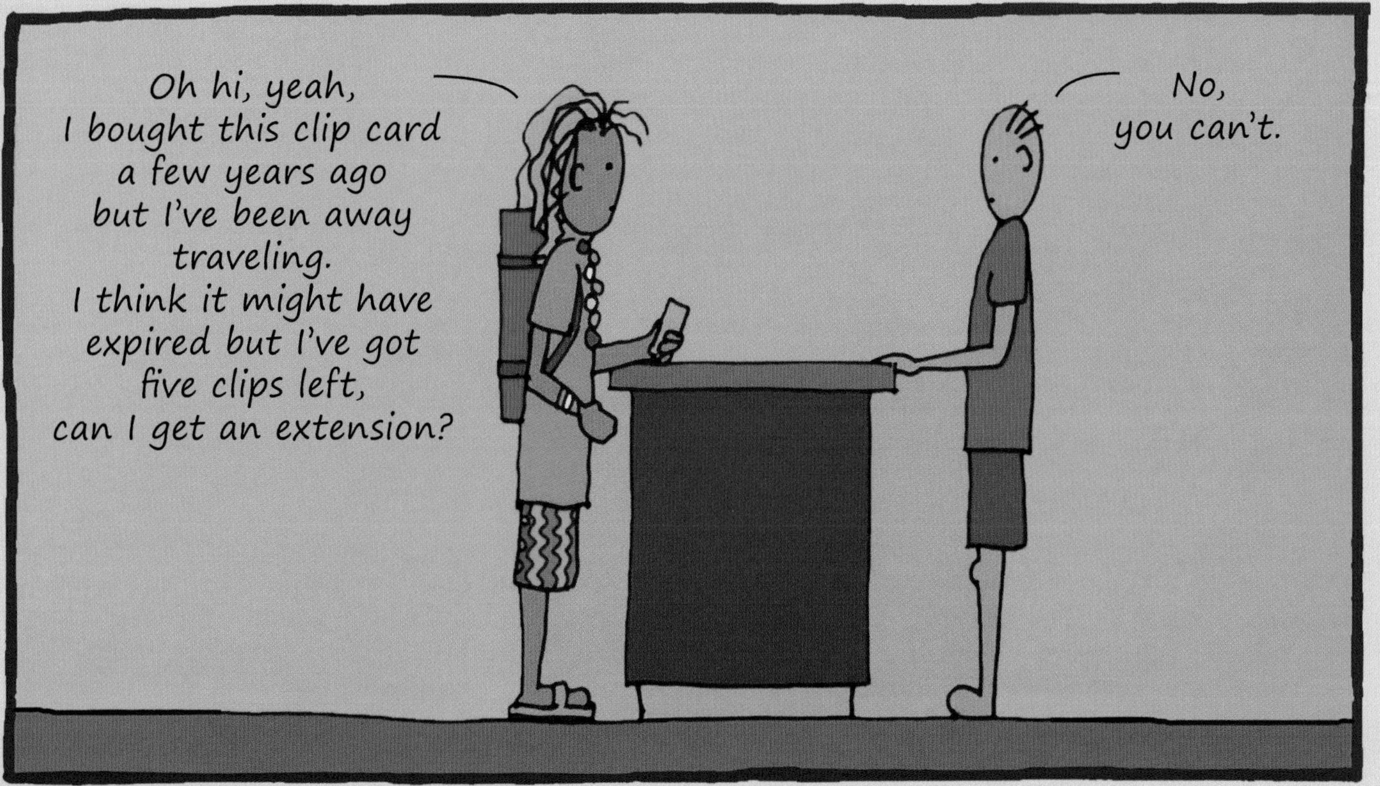

Oh hi, yeah,
I bought this clip card
a few years ago
but I've been away
traveling.
I think it might have
expired but I've got
five clips left,
can I get an extension?
No,
you can't.

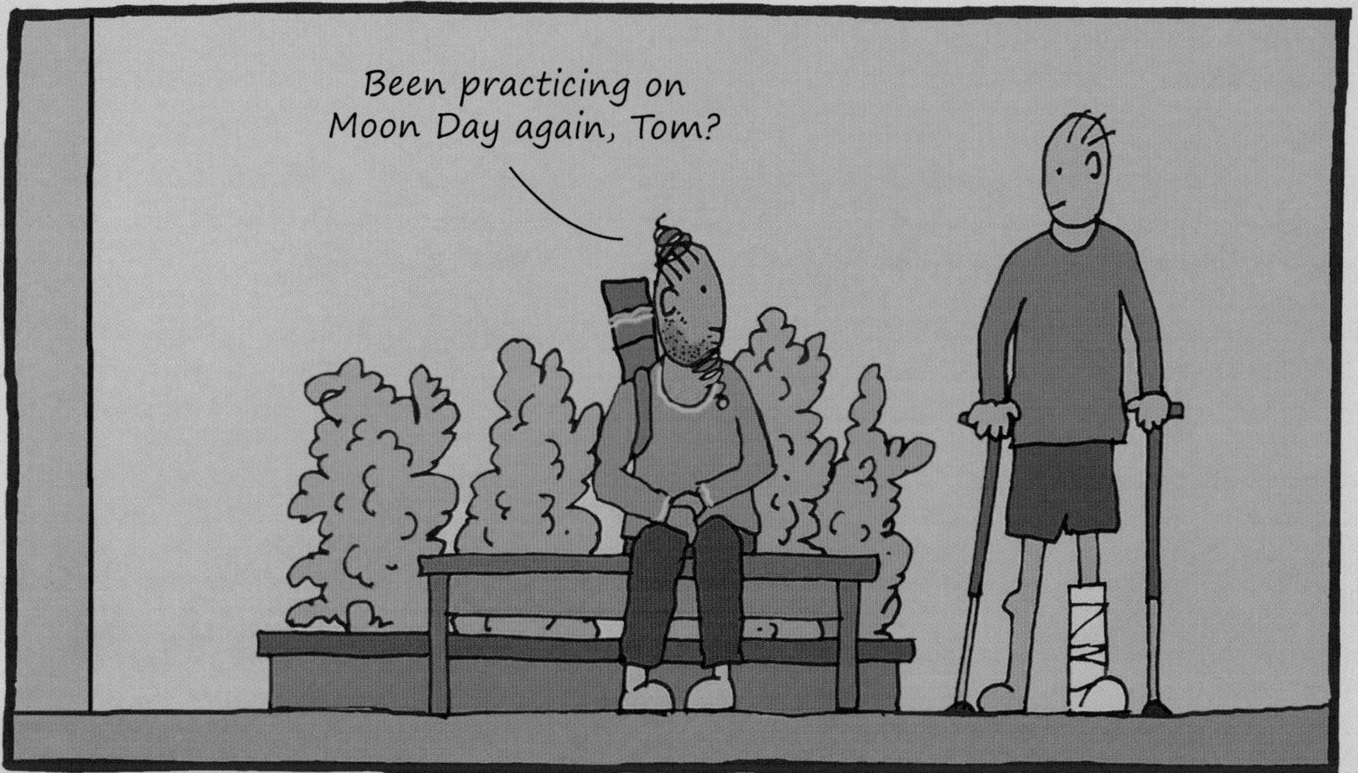
Been practicing on
Moon Day again, Tom?

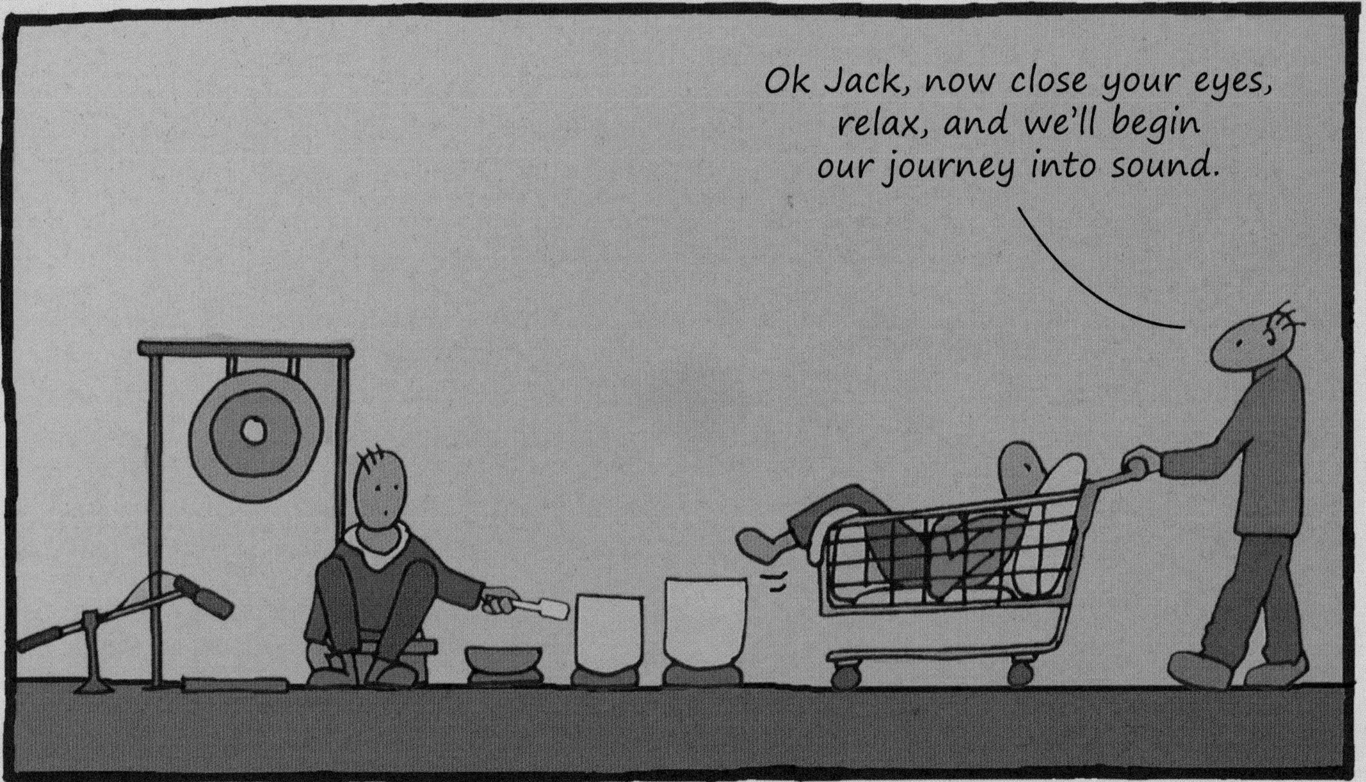
Ok Jack, now close your eyes,
relax, and we'll begin
our journey into sound.

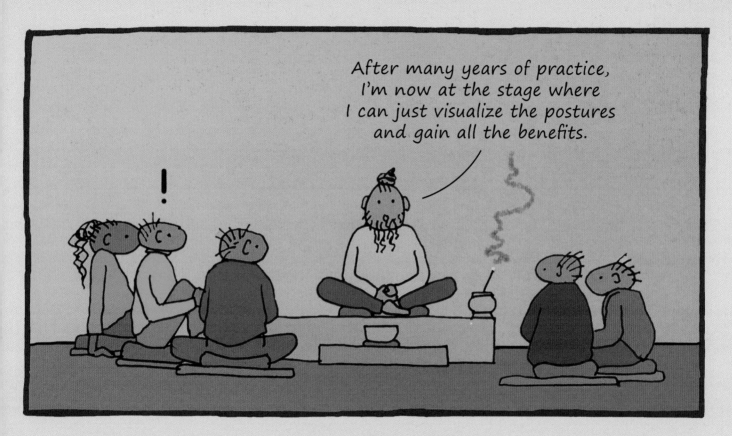

William could suddenly smell something in the room other than incense.

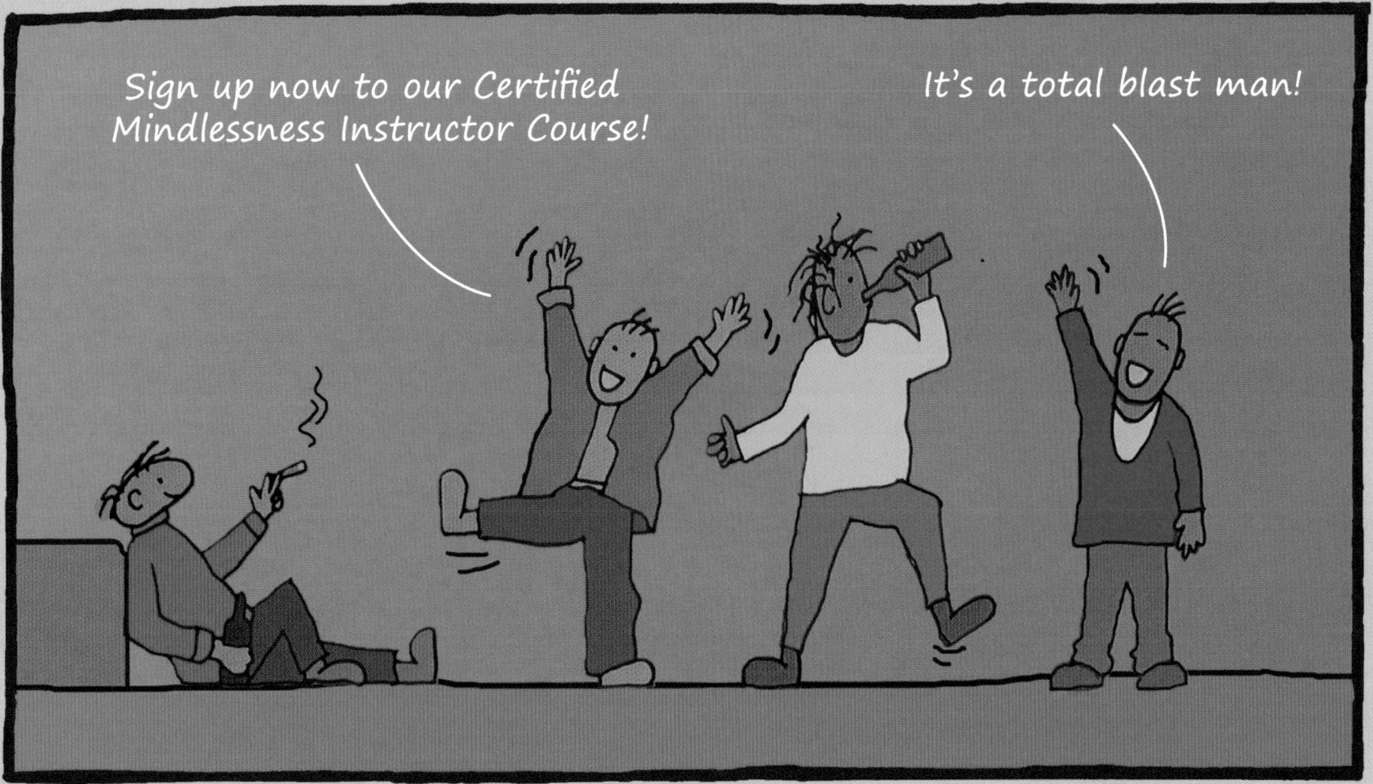
Sign up now to our Certified Mindlessness Instructor Course!
It's a total blast man!

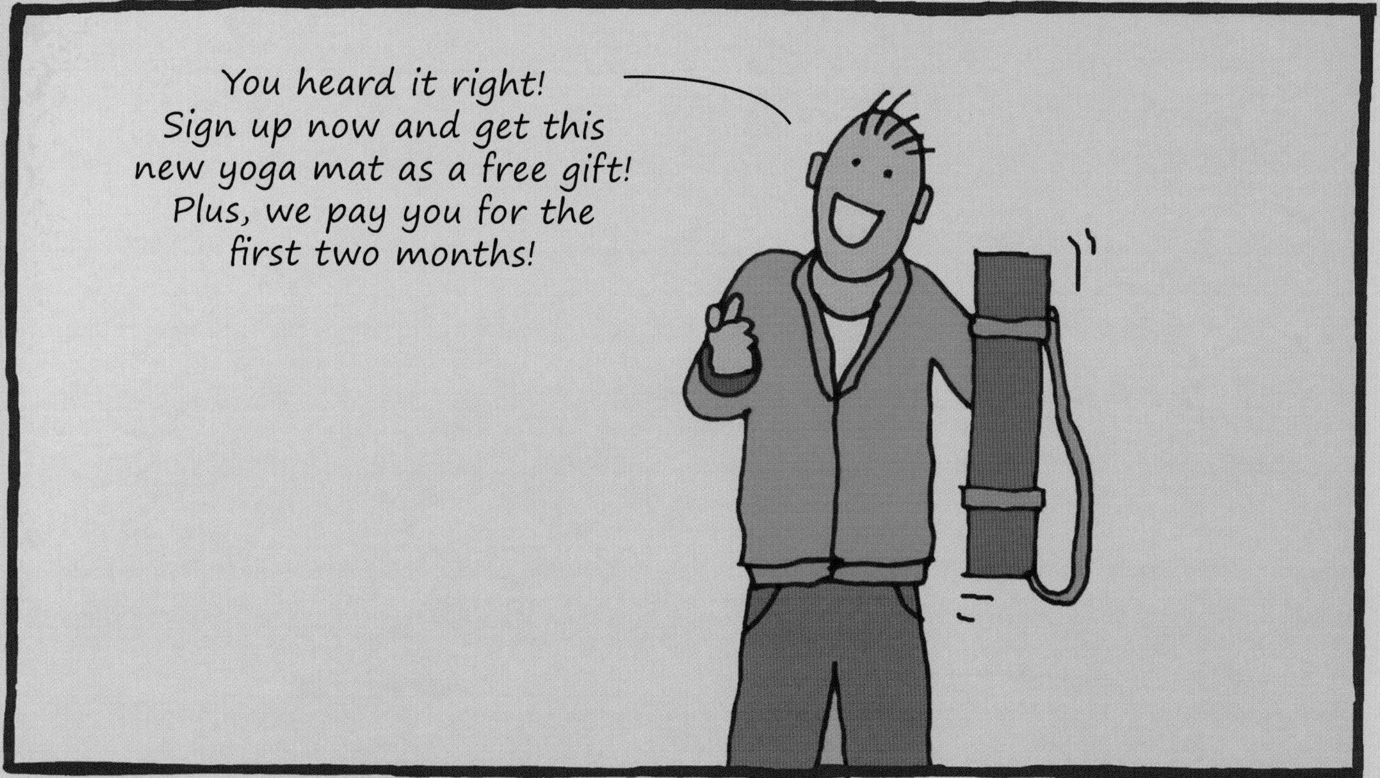
You heard it right!
Sign up now and get this
new yoga mat as a free gift!
Plus, we pay you for the
first two months!

Next-level marketing.

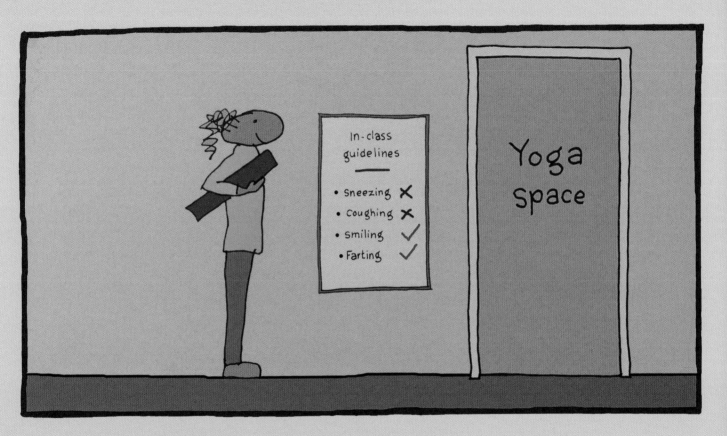

Carol was on board with the new COVID guidelines.

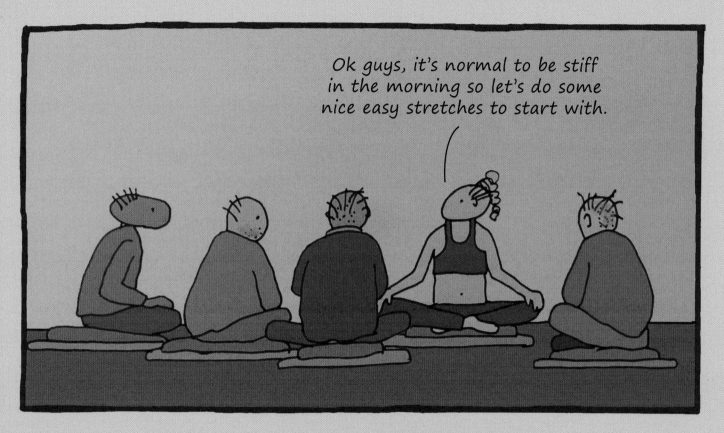

Sarah hadn't really thought through her opening line
to the morning session of "Yoga for guys."

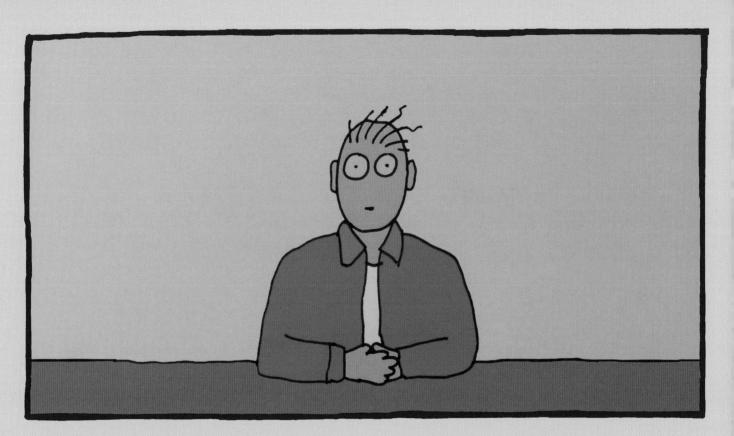

Four days later and Robert was still enjoying the effects
of the Hypnotic Shamanic Drumming Intensive.

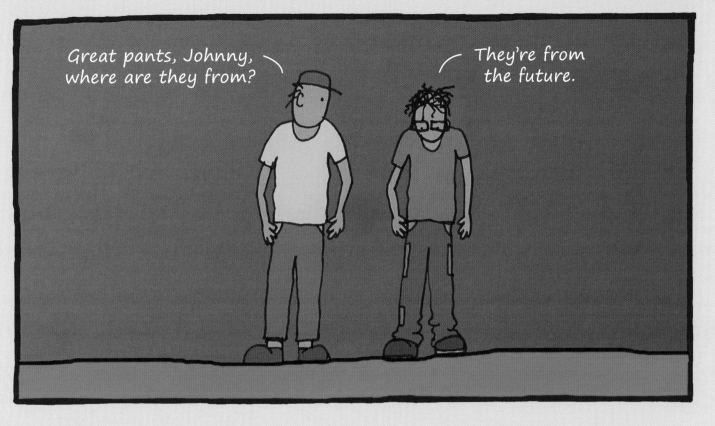

There was no such thing as a normal conversation with Cosmic Johnny.

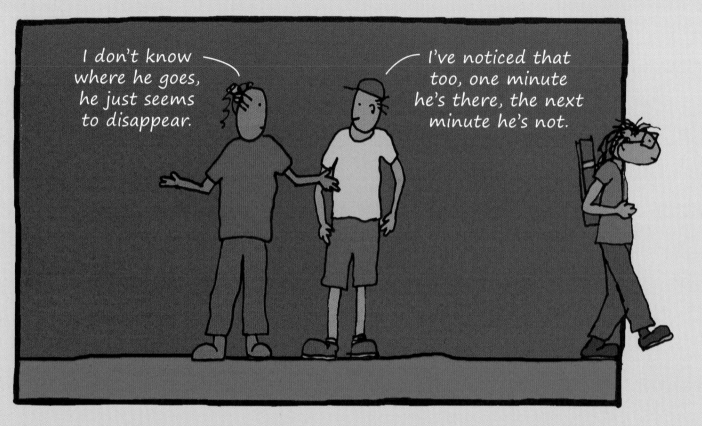

Through deep meditation, Cosmic Johnny had developed
the ability to step into the fourth dimension.

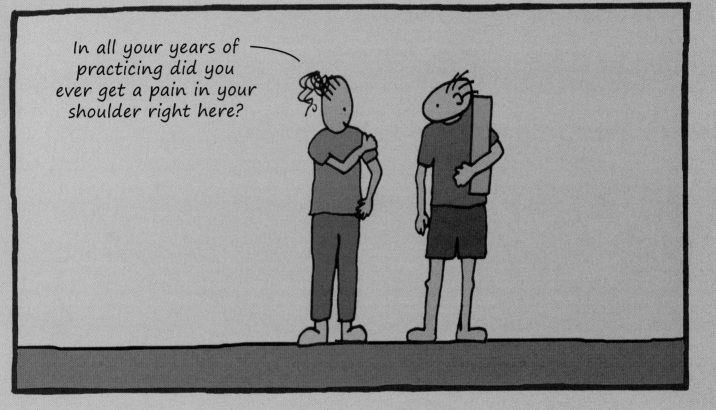

After teaching the class and bidding goodnight to all the students, there was one final question for teacher Simon.

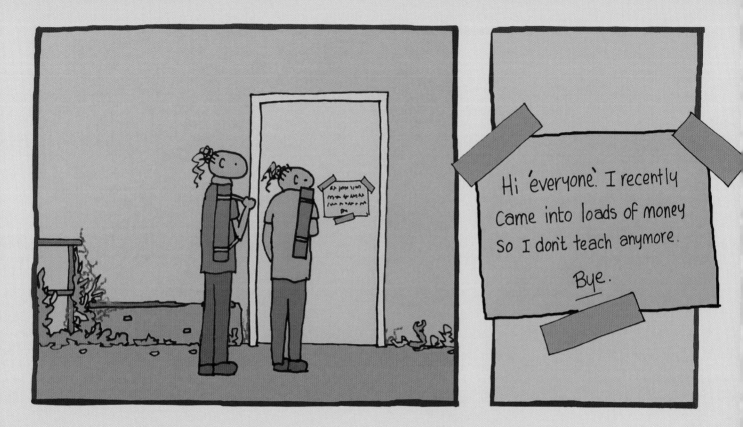

When the two regulars showed up for the morning Hatha class,
there was a note stuck on the door.

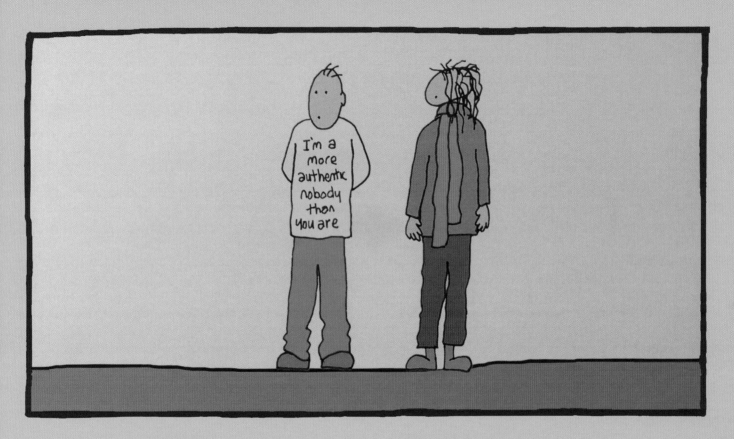

Subtle competition during silent meditation retreats.

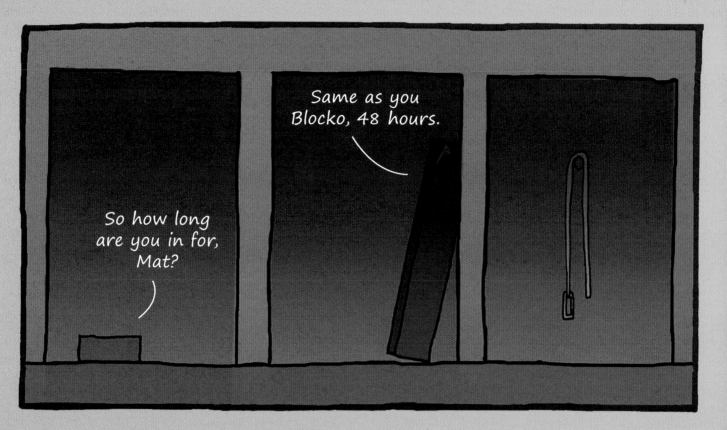

Even yoga equipment found itself in quarantine during the Corona pandemic.

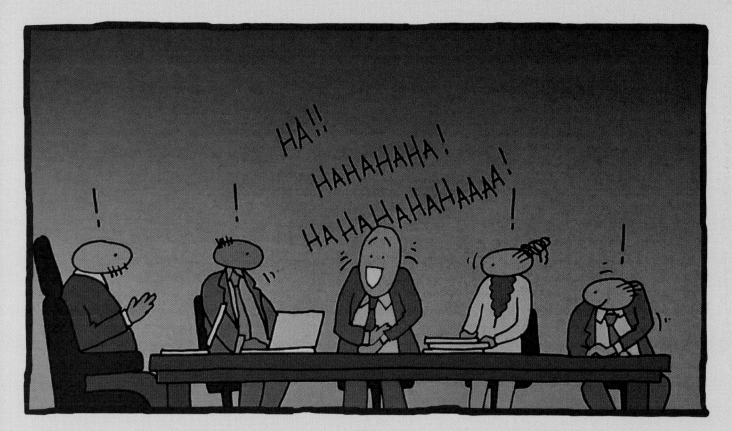

After the weekend Laughter Yoga Intensive, Julian just couldn't hold it together during the office Monday morning briefing.

A common experience usually occurring somewhere
around mid to advanced asana.

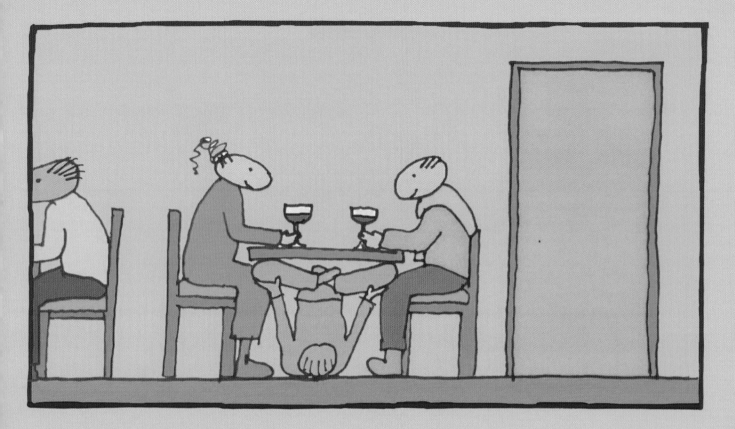

Creative ways yoga teachers can supplement their income in difficult times:
1. Hire yourself out as an Organic Table.

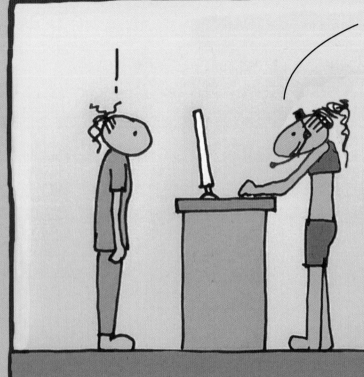

Sally had a two-point plan for stress reduction:
1. Simplify her life. 2. Start doing yoga.

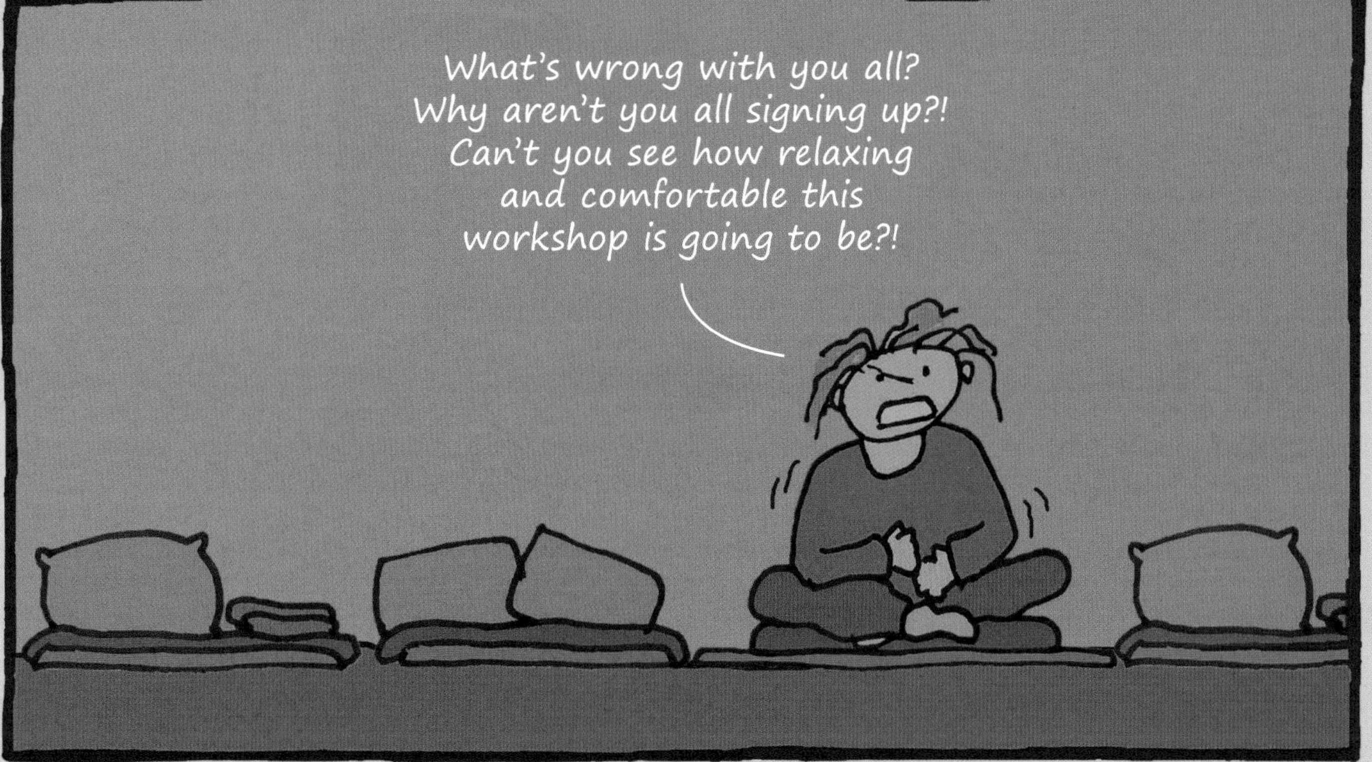
What's wrong with you all?
Why aren't you all signing up?!
Can't you see how relaxing
and comfortable this
workshop is going to be?!

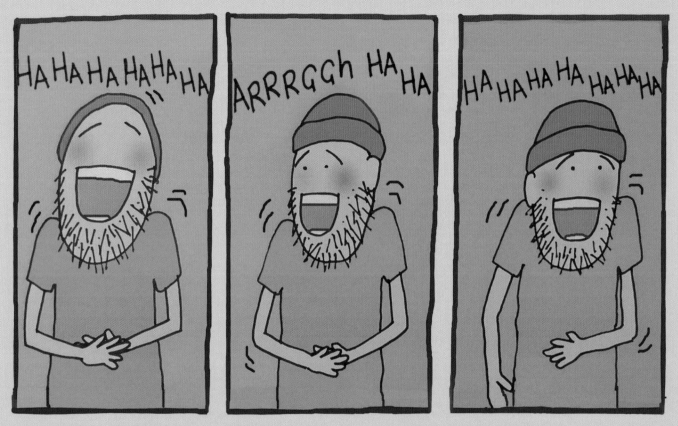

After a brief introduction to the Laughter Yoga workshop,
teacher Benjamin got straight to it.

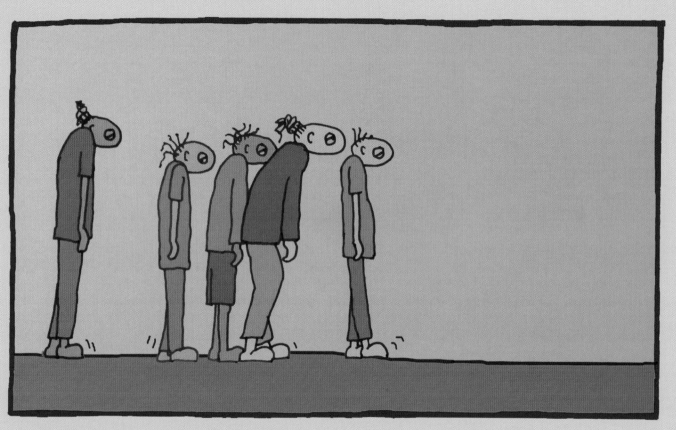

Feeling the full effects of Level 1, the participants now shuffled their way to Level 2 of the "Relax and spoil yourself" workshop.

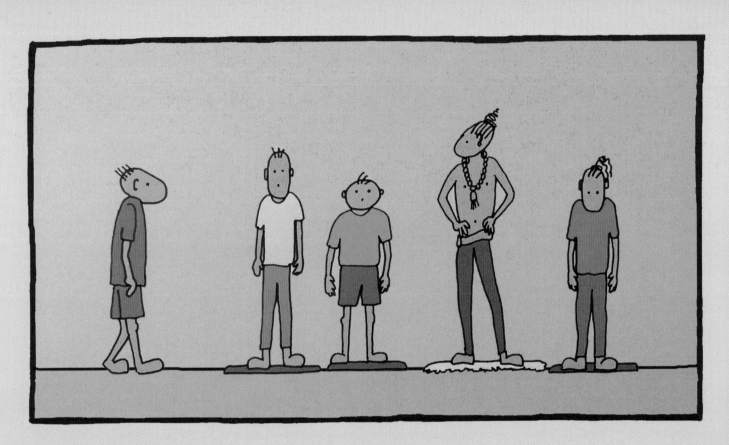

Upon entering the class,
teacher Dave could instantly sense an oncoming ego clash.

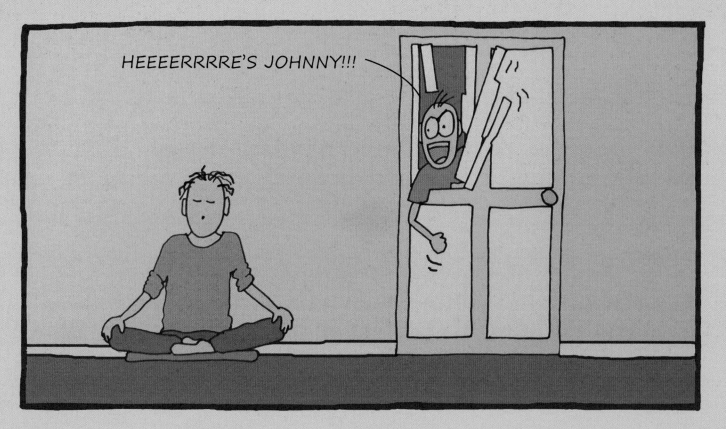

One thing was for sure, folks had very different ways
of handling stress during lockdown.

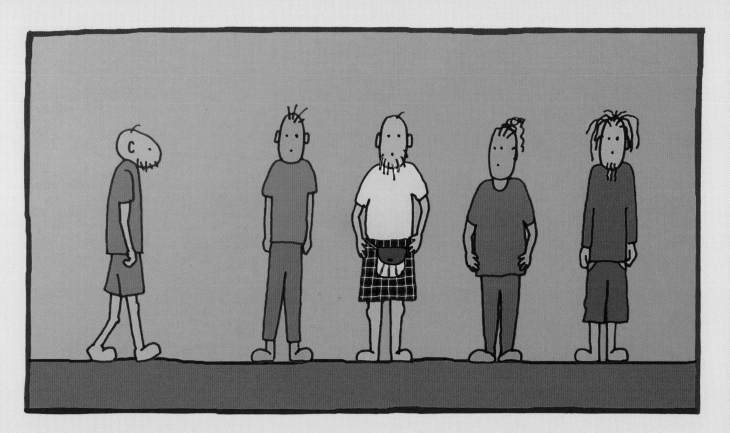

Teacher Mike could foresee some potential issues with John's outfit when it came to the headstand and shoulderstand.

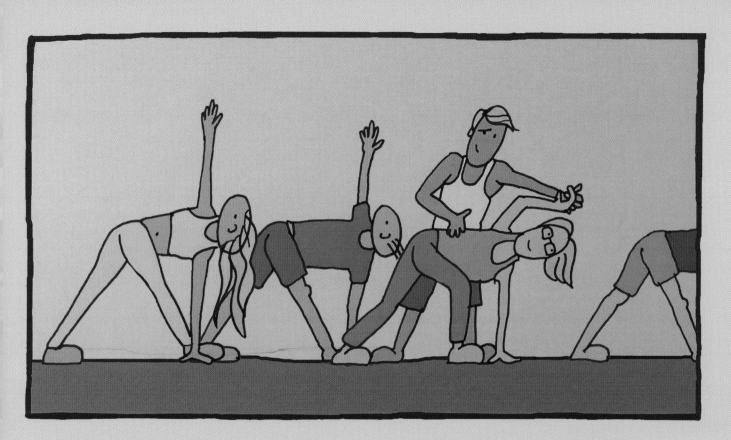

In Kyle's classes, Susanna would purposely do the poses incorrectly just to get those extra adjustments.

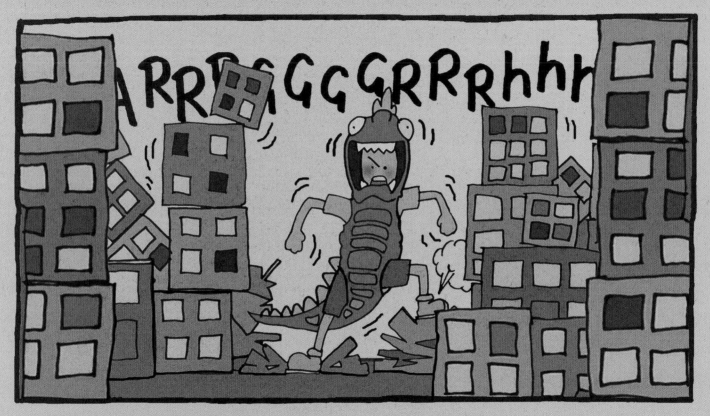

The revolutionary new stress therapy involved dressing up in a rubber Godzilla outfit and then going completely bonkers in a warehouse full of cardboard boxes painted up to look like buildings.

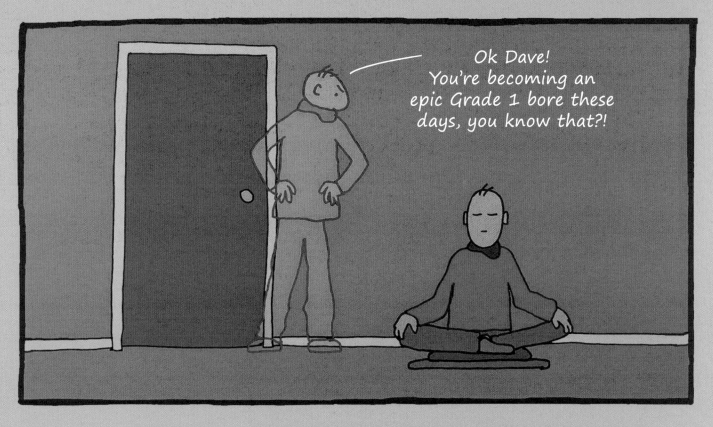

Dave's ego was becoming more and more concerned.

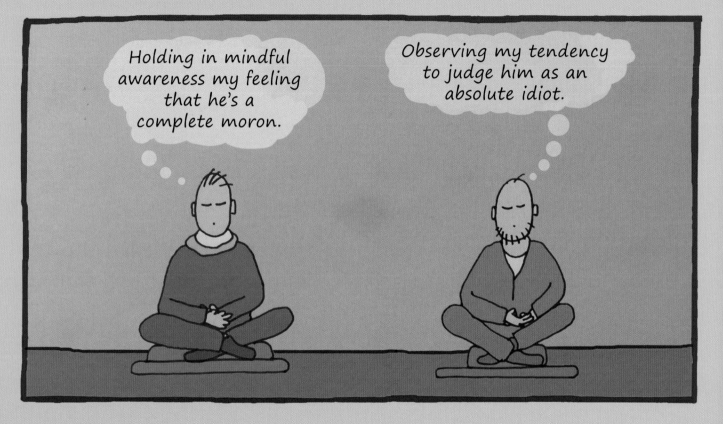

Conflict between participants
on Mindfulness and Meditation retreats.

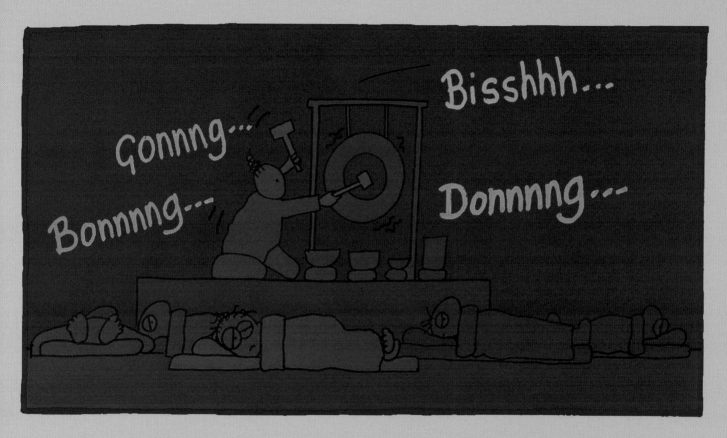

By the time 4 a.m. arrived, Rachel wasn't quite as convinced about the "bliss" element of the "All Night Gong Bliss" event.

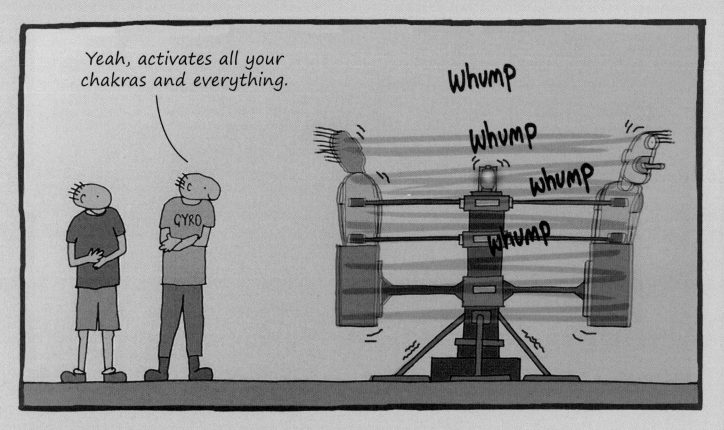

Colin wasn't entirely convinced
by the sales demo for Gyro-Yoga.

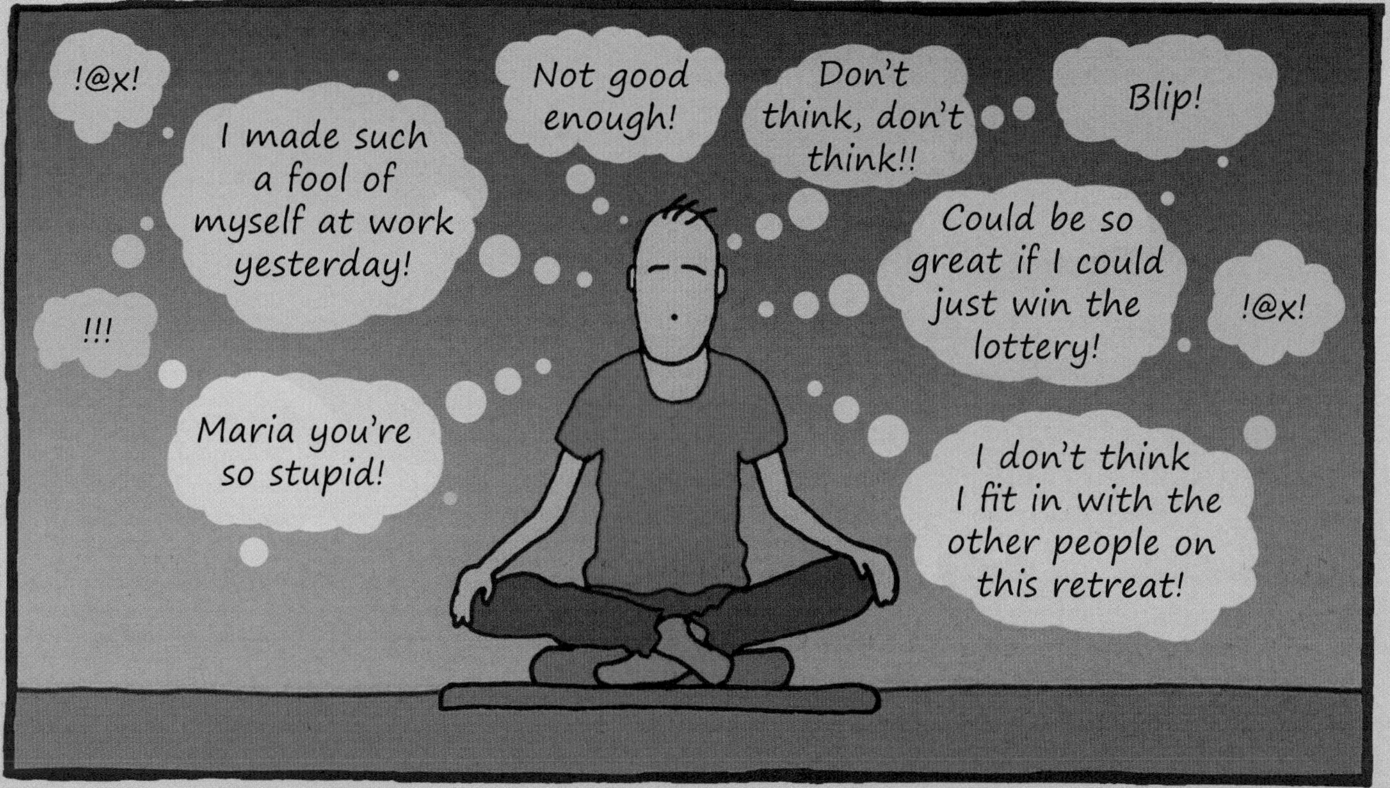
!@x!
I made such a fool of myself at work yesterday!
!!!
Maria you're so stupid!
Not good enough!
Don't think, don't think!!
Blip!
Could be so great if I could just win the lottery!
!@x!
I don't think I fit in with the other people on this retreat!

Meditative Bliss.

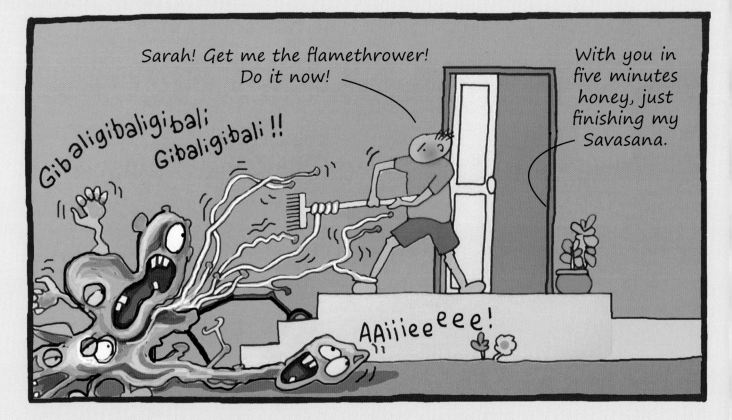

Sarah never rushed her Savasana,
even when things became stressful.

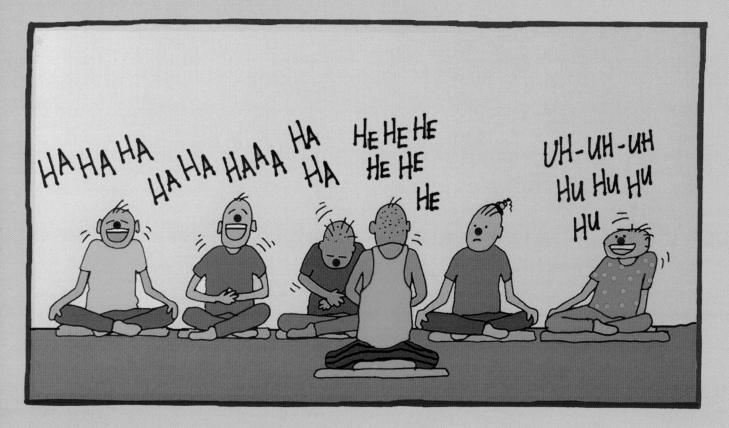

Penelope had to concede,
she just didn't find Laughter Yoga funny.

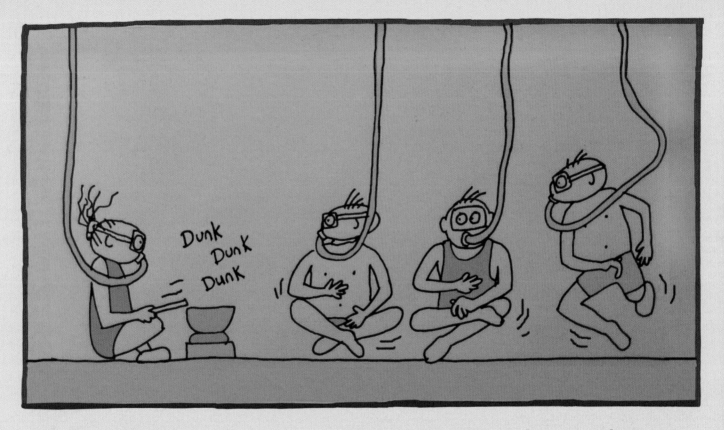

Teacher Nora had the idea of doing an Underwater Gong Bath session, but pretty quickly they all agreed that the gongs just didn't sound the same under water.

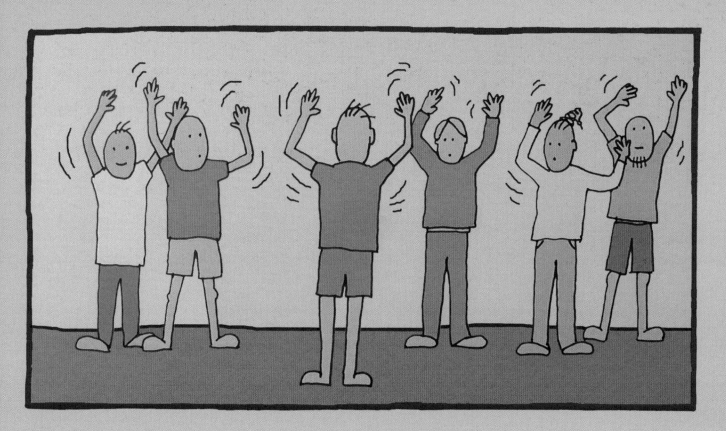

Teacher Henry was so nervous on his teaching debut that he couldn't actually speak, all he could do was wave his arms and everyone followed.

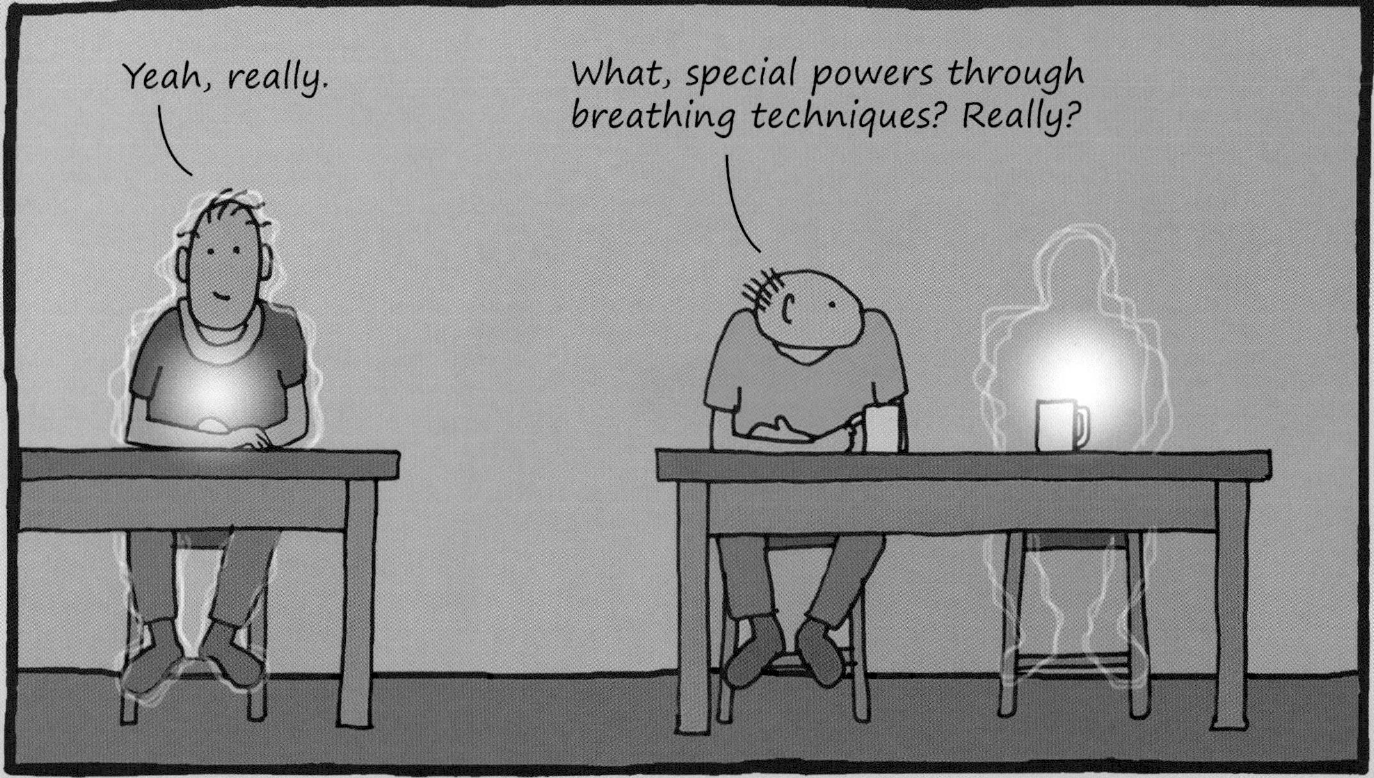
Yeah, really.
What, special powers through breathing techniques? Really?

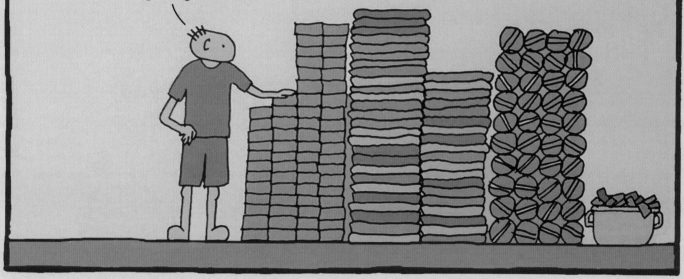

Setting things up in Charlie's Restorative Yoga sessions could take a while.

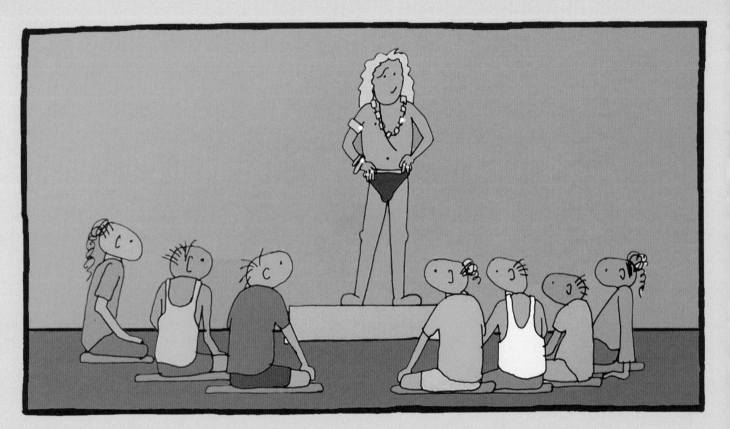

A number of the participants were not entirely convinced that Nigel was the right teacher to lead the "Transcend your ego" workshop.

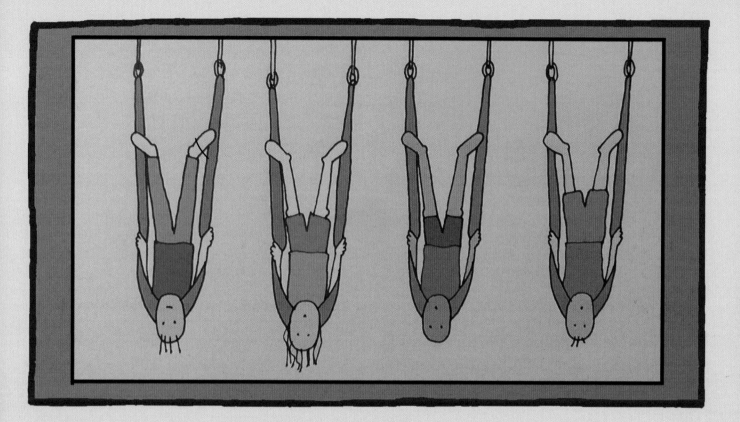

Carol had to admit that the new photo for Ariel Yoga sessions looked more like a promo for a horror movie.

So in today's video, I'm going to focus on exercises that tone and improve our digestive system.

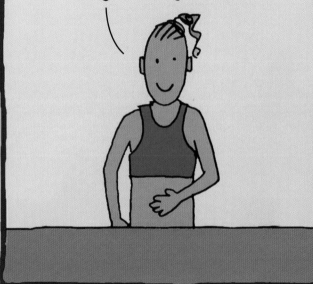

So that we can then stuff our faces with cakes and chocolates and all the happy foods! Yeeeaahhhhh!!!

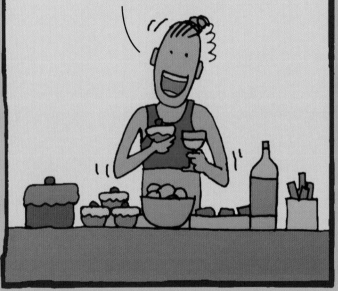

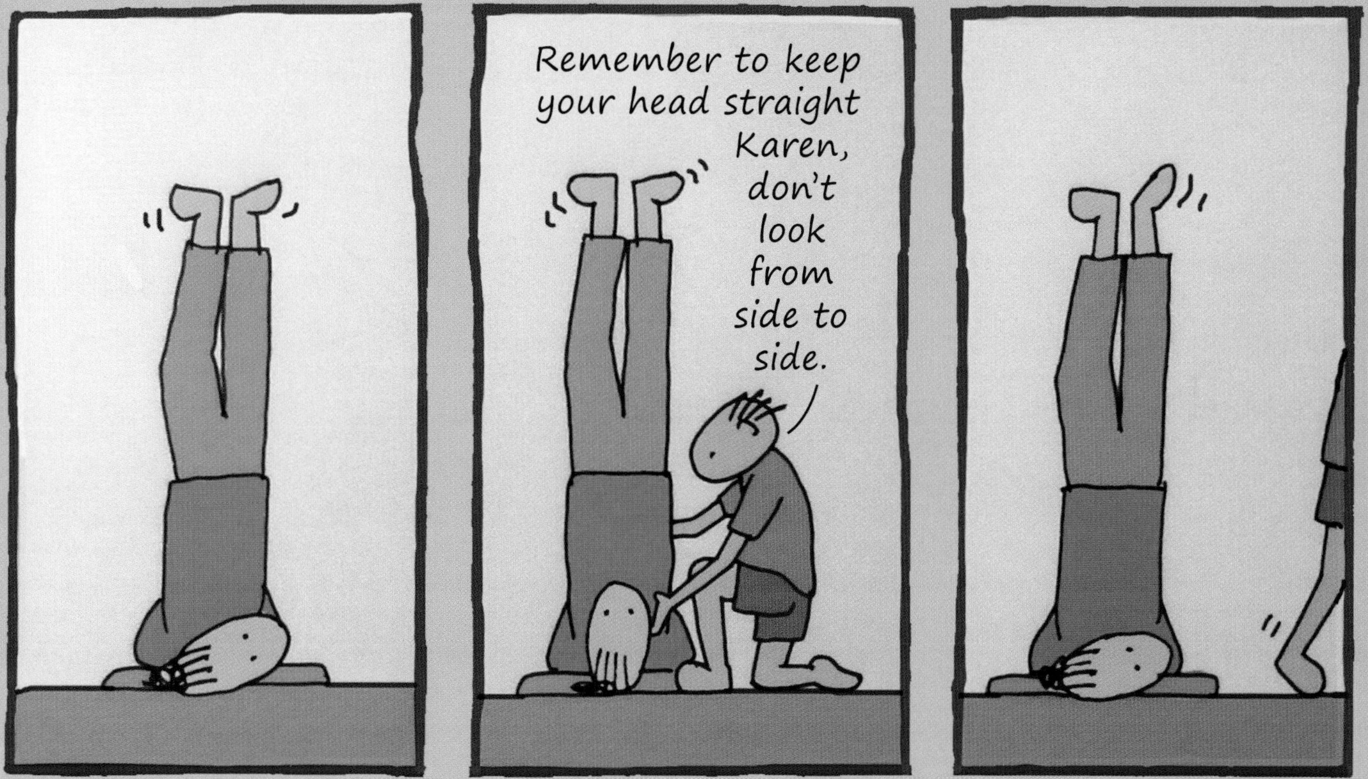
Remember to keep your head straight Karen, don't look from side to side.

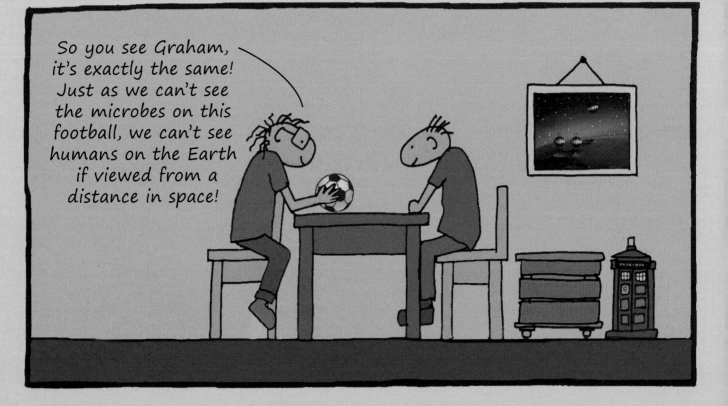

After a week of intense fasting and meditation, Cosmic Johnny was really unloading some epic insight onto his best friend Graham.

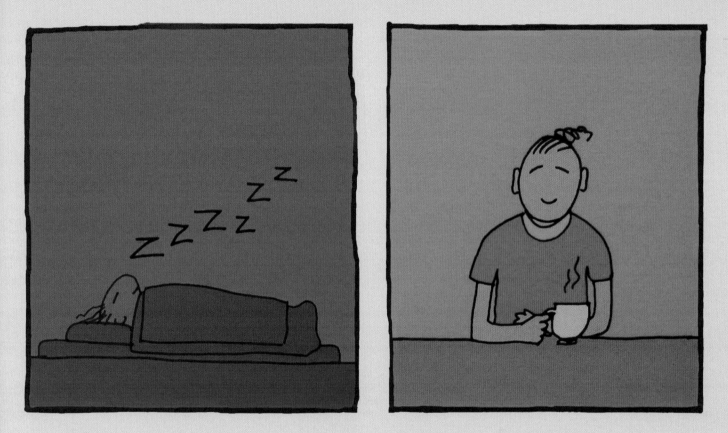

Lily was dedicated to her morning yoga sessions, which typically consisted of a 45-minute session of Savasana followed by one or two cups of freshly brewed coffee.

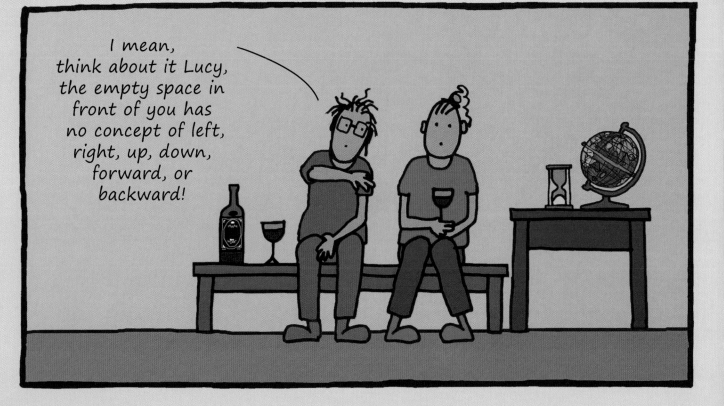

After his third glass of wine,
Cosmic Johnny was rolling.

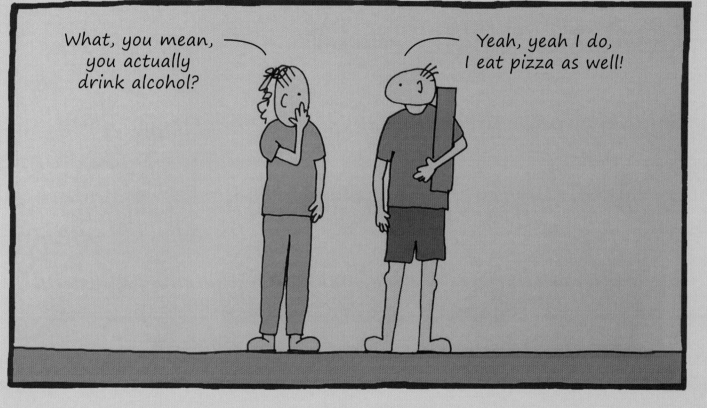

Scarlett was genuinely shocked to find out that teacher Charles was not in actual fact a purified being from another dimension.

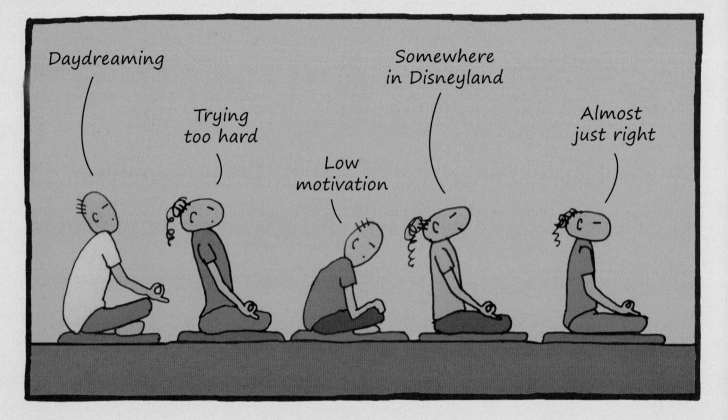

Yogic sitting positions explained.

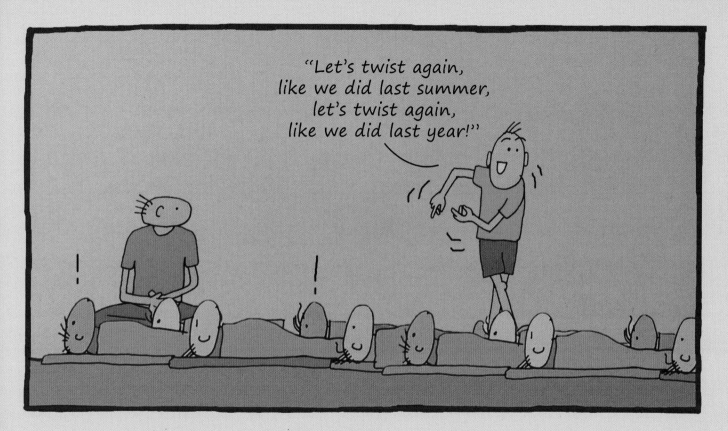

Teacher Mark thought it was a great idea for Nigel to perform a relaxing song during Savasana, but it quickly became apparent that they had very different ideas about what constituted "relaxing."

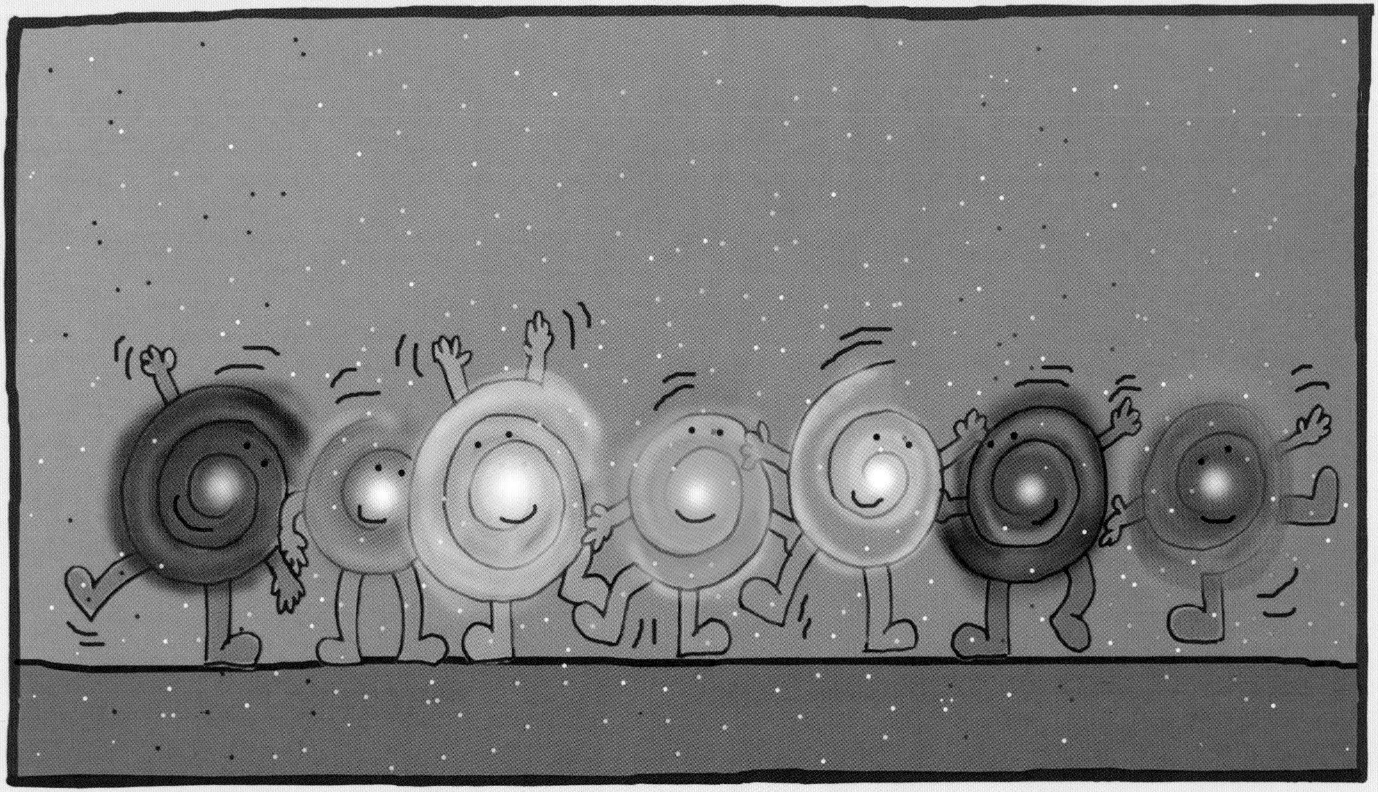

Chakra Dance.